SPIRITUAL AWAKENING ACADEMY

# THIRD EYE AWAKENING

*Guided Meditation to Open Your Third Eye.*

*Psychic Abilities for Beginners, Mind Power, Intuition, Empath, Healing Mediumship, Mindfulness, Aura reading, Yoga, Chakra and Reiki*

By **Spiritual Awakening Academy**

## Table of Contents

- INTRODUCTION — 3
- CHAPTER 1: WHAT IS THE THIRD EYE? — 5
- CHAPTER 2: HOW TO OPEN YOUR THIRD EYE — 10
- CHAPTER 3: TECHNIQUES TO AWAKEN THE THIRD EYE CHAKRA — 21
- CHAPTER 4: GUIDED DAY MEDITATIONS TO AWAKEN THE THIRD EYE — 39
- CHAPTER 5: THE POWERS OF AN OPEN THIRD EYE
- CHAPTER 6: PSYCHIC ABILITIES — 72
- CHAPTER 7: PSYCHIC AWARENESS — 89
- CHAPTER 8: EXERCISES FOR AWAKENING YOUR INNER SPIRIT — 92
- CHAPTER 9: PINEAL GLAND ACTIVATION AND CHAKRAS — 98
- CHAPTER 10: HOW TO MAINTAIN THE HEALTH OF YOUR THIRD EYE OVER TIME? — 113
- CHAPTER 11: COMMON MISTAKES PEOPLE MAKE TRYING TO ACTIVATE THE THIRD EYE — 137
- CONCLUSION — 143

## Introduction

The third eye has been a mystical concept for centuries. Very few people have known this power and they kept it a secret for very long. It has widely been a misrepresented and misinterpreted concept. Opening the third eye is no magic. It will not happen through some gadgets or accessories. It is a journey within. You will have to undertake it alone. You can open your third eye with devotion, willpower, and meditation. It is possible and thousands of people are doing it. The best thing about this process is not only the result but the journey in itself is also very beautiful.

The third eye is the most eloquent source of intuitive wisdom. A power only possessed by the yogis, psychics and fortune tellers in the past. If you meditate and open your third eye then you can get insights, prior warnings of danger and high level of intelligence at the time. The keyword to achieve this objective is meditation.

The Ajna chakra or the third eye is located in the pineal gland. For centuries, the occultists and the spiritual masters have called it the 'seat of the soul'. Once you are able to open your third eye, the difference between the truth and reality becomes crystal clear. You are able to connect yourself with the higher energy field and feel what is impossible to feel in any other way. Getting very high intuitive power is another aspect of it. You become highly aware and establish a connection with your surroundings. Your gut feeling gets stronger. Your sixth sense starts working predominantly.

The third eye awakens your inner self. You easily establish a connection with your surroundings. The reason for most of the sorrows in our lives is our discontent. The new awakening introduces you to a world of new realization. Your perception of good and bad will change. You can see things deeply and not from the superficial level. You react differently and in a much-matured way. This is a completely new feeling. It is like an intellectual looking at the immature quarrels of the kids.

## Chapter 1: What Is the Third Eye?

The third eye is perhaps the most mysterious, powerful organ in the body. At about the size of a walnut, this tiny organ located in the brain has eluded mystics and scientists alike for centuries. In this chapter, we will discuss the myths and perceived powers of this amazing gland, and what has emerged in the scientific community that supports these ideas.

First, let's go back centuries ago. Thousands of years ago, the exact year doesn't matter, people across the globe searched for answers to their most burning question: What are we on this earth for? People sought far and wide, experimenting with different lifestyles and means to connect with a higher power, only to come up short. What they found is that all of the answers to their questions, as individual as they were, lay right inside their own mind. The key to life was reaching deep within themselves to find the answers they sought. The thought across many cultures, most isolated from one another, is that our third eye is the window to our inner selves, our soul, and our connection with the energy and power of the universe. Creating a deeper understanding of this small area, located on the forehead, just between the eyes seems to be like opening a door into another world. Truly, it is.

The idea that each of us has a soul or an inner self is certainly nothing new either. Our outer self is our worldly skin, what we present in a physical way to others and to the world. We can tangibly see the outer self of everyone around us, and it doesn't change too much. Think of your inner self as a ball of energy, bright and ever-changing that is driving our body forward.

It is this energy that connects us with the energy of the universe. Consider yourself just a small bit of energy in a much larger matrix of energy that creates our known universe. All of the energy is connected, and should you choose to be wholly part of it, you can benefit from its positivity and force. Being in a good flow of energy manifests itself as leading a life that is fulfilling and purposeful.

Let's look at the third eye from a more scientific perspective. The third eye is actually called the pineal gland, a small organ located at the very top of the spine as it enters the brain. It is distinctly in the center of the brain, between the left and right hemispheres. From the outside, it would be dead center between, and just above the eyes. An air of excitement and mystery surrounded this organ as soon as it was discovered. This tiny thing must be important. Otherwise, it wouldn't be tucked away so safely within the brain. What could it be?

The pineal gland is primarily responsible for the production of melatonin, a hormone that is required for regulating our circadian rhythm. It is this vigilance of light and dark that allows us to fall asleep and wake up in a normal pattern. Disruptions in melatonin cause sleep disruption, insomnia, narcolepsy and general fatigue.

Another curious thing about the pineal gland is that it creates and houses a chemical that is known to cause so-called hallucinations.

Dimethyltryptamine (DMT), is naturally produced in the body and can be compared to psychedelic drugs like acid, a man-made version. DMT in large amounts causes the mind to slip into a trance-like state, and vivid imagery occurs. This chemical is released in small doses when we sleep, creating dreams.

For those who partake in the use of psychedelic drugs often report being reborn, awakened into a new life by the experience. This type of drug has been used for centuries in Native American and South American cultures (along with many more) for spiritual practice and connection with the gods. It is hard to ignore the fact that entering such a state opens the mind and has the potential to connect our inner selves with a higher energy. Could this be the key to knowing our inner selves?

Even though the pineal gland is located smack dab in the center of the brain, our inner selves, and our brains don't always communicate with each other. The brain is a strong organ which is driven by organic, analytical thought. Its job is to take in information from our environment, process it, and understand it. The brain is the computer that recognizes what color something is but does not necessarily put deeper thought into it.

Although that example is oversimplified a bit, it is our inner selves that really attach meaning and understanding to things. When the brain and soul are not aligned with each other, it can cause our brain to react without guidance and wisdom of the bigger picture. So, we are required to get in touch with our inner self more often to lead a life with infinite wisdom and guidance.

Awakening our third eye without the help of medications is certainly possible as well. There are many practices we can do on a regular basis that help open the mind and deepen the connection between our inner selves and our analytical brains. The world we live in constantly forces us to work against the better judgment of our inner selves, and so the number of people being spiritually guided are the minority.

What most people don't realize, however, is that they are living in a fallacy of a world in which their physical bodies and analytical minds are at one. The mind and body are disposable, and what is left after we are gone is our inner selves, our spirit, to become connected, once again, with the energy of the universe. We must do the best we can to live out tangible lives through the needs and desires of our spirit, and not let the worldly needs of the body take hold. Our souls do not need money or power, they need love and understanding. Our time here on earth could be made so much happier and healthier by following the guidance of our inner spirit. Getting connected with our third eye is the key to all of it.

## Chapter 2: How To Open Your Third Eye

Opening your third eye takes time and practice. While you may have an experience, such as during meditation, where you feel a huge rush of awakening, it will not be fully awakened by one experience. Rather, the awakening is a process and you must take your time and commit to it if you are going to experience a full awakening.

Beginning with meditation is a great way to start opening your third eye, but there are additional ways that you can open it as well. In this chapter, we are going to explore the other ways that you can open your third eye, in addition to meditation. Some of these are practices that you must set aside time for, while others are ones that you can use in your regular daily life. As you are using these practices, it is important to understand that your third eye awakening will be a very spiritual and individual process, but having it in an awakened state means that you are going to integrate it into your daily life. Awakening your third eye should not consume all of your time and result in you doing nothing but focusing on the awakened state of your third eye. Rather, you should set aside some time but otherwise focus on leading your life as you normally would. As your third eye awakens, you will notice differences about yourself that stem from this awakening process. However, you should continue leading your daily life and allowing these changes to naturally integrate, rather than forcing them. Anything forced is not natural, and therefore may inhibit the opening process for your third eye.

Learn to Silence Your Mind

In addition to proper meditation, practice silencing your mind. When we go about our daily lives, there tends to be a lot of chatter and noise in our minds that can keep us constantly distracted and focused on everything except what we are doing. A great way to support your third eye awakening is to learn to silence your mind and focus only on the task at hand. When you do, your mind will be focused, and the background will be silenced. It is typically within' these silences that the third eye and our psychic abilities will kick in and take place.

While it is impossible to entirely stop thinking, you should stay very intentional with your thinking process and focus specifically on what you need to be thinking about depending on what you are physically doing. The third eye chakra tends to "activate" and work during the "in between" times that take place between thoughts and experiences. Therefore, if you want to intentionally activate it, you need to intentionally set aside space for these in-between moments to happen. When you do, make sure that you are paying attention and are aware of when they happen so that you can focus on them and practice strengthening your ability to activate them whenever you desire.

Practice Tuning In

When you feel or hear something coming from your intuition, take the time to acknowledge it, and then actually listen to it. Do whatever it says, and then notice what happens as a result. In many instances life becomes easier, a hazard is avoided, we recognize or learn something we may have missed, or things are otherwise "better" overall. Sometimes these realizations may not be as obvious, but they do exist. Learning to tune into your intuition means you are learning to acknowledge and give credit to your third eye. And, as the saying says "where your attention goes, energy flows" which means that if you are intentionally listening to your third eye and your intuition, it will continue speaking to you. The more you tune in and listen, the better your "relationship" or connection will be, and the better results you will get from tuning in.

Explore Your Natural Creativity

Our creative sides are largely linked to our third eye. Those who are highly creative tend to be very creative, or interested in increasing their creative abilities. If you want to connect closer to your third eye, practice embracing your creativity and letting it free. Even if you don't think you are a good artist or you are inexperienced with various art forms, practice them anyway. Let your imagination take over and create anything that comes to mind. Don't hold expectations of what it should or shouldn't look like, just create. You will find that when you do this, your third eye chakra will feel more enhanced naturally. Remember, your third eye is also your "mind's eye" which means that it is your imagination. When you create from your imagination, you are directly creating from your third eye. It can be an incredible experience alongside your awakening process.

Take Time to Ground Yourself

## THIRD EYE AWAKENING

Your third eye can take you into the spiritual realm through your mind's eye and your intuition, and when you are not careful it can affect your ability to stay grounded. When you are working with your third eye, you should be simultaneously working with your root chakra and grounding yourself. You can do this by meditating on your root chakra and imagine actual etheric roots connecting you to the center of the Earth. This is a great way to counterbalance your third eye and keep you rooted while also allowing you to explore your awakening.

When you don't take the time to root yourself, you can experience what is known as "overstimulation", which means your third eye is working more than your other chakras. This can lead to stress, discomfort, being overwhelmed, and many other unwanted experiences. When the process of awakening becomes uncomfortable, people are more likely to avoid it and therefore they can find themselves not wanting to further their awakening. Furthermore, they might shut their eye out of fear and have difficulty wanting to return to the awakening process at any point in the future. To avoid being overwhelmed and the discomfort, make sure you are always focusing on grounding yourself. If you are not a major fan of meditation, you can also allow your bare feet to connect directly to the Earth, as this is a great physical grounding process.

Exercise Your Third Eye

Exercising your third eye is a great way to help support its opening. It also increases your strength and abilities, meaning you will have an easier time keeping it open, using it on a regular basis, and activating your psychic abilities at any time which you desire. The following are great exercises you can practice to help you support your third eye opening.

One great way is to do meditations that involve all of the chakras. Similar to how it is important to ground and focus on your root chakra, you should also focus on strengthening your other chakras, too. While you may wish to primarily focus on strengthening and growing your abilities with them one at a time, it is important that you continue to give focus to each of them. When one or two chakras become overstimulated from being used more than the others, it can create a spiritual imbalance that can create unwanted side effects for the individual. A great meditation is to lay down and meditate, then imagine your chakras one at a time. Start with your root chakra and work your way up to your crown chakra. As you go, imagine each one shining brighter and brighter until it is shining its brightest. You can also imagine them spinning clockwise, as they are a fluid energy that moves, they do not simply beam like a lamp, but rather swirl like a whirlpool.

Another great way to work with your third eye is to do dream work. Using lucid dreaming meditations, and practicing dream interpretation are both great ways to practice dream work. Lucid dreaming is typically completed using meditations, where you allow yourself to go into a dream state and then you mentally control yourself in the dream state. It allows you to be in control of your dream, rather than your dream be in control like they typically are. Dream interpretation itself requires you to allow the dream to flow naturally, and then you interpret it upon waking up. The best way to do this is to write about your dream in the moments after you have woken up. You can then interpret them on your own, or purchase a dream interpretation journal to help you interpret different elements within' the dream.

Allowing your imagination to flow naturally and on its own is another great way to play with your third eye. Practice sitting in a meditative state, and then let your imagination flow. Just follow it anywhere it goes. During this type of meditation, there is no need to draw your attention back to any particular place, you can simply let it go to wherever it desires to be. You can also allow your imagination to flow while you are creating such as through drawing, writing, pottery, or other crafts. Allowing your meditation to take charge and faithfully following it can help you feel more connected to your third eye, and can help support its awakening.

Intuition lead breaks are another great way to strengthen your third eye. Like with playing with your imagination, you are letting your intuition lead the way. This means that you go anywhere and do anything that your intuition is telling you to. So, if your intuition tells you to go sit by a particular tree in a certain park and look in a certain direction, you do it. When you follow your intuition this way, you leave yourself open to receiving mental "downloads" that are often filled with information that can be beneficial to your present state. You might learn something about yourself, be guided to take a specific action in a certain situation, or otherwise feel lead to do something. All of these stem from your third eye guidance and should be honored when you experience them during this time. If you will recall, honoring your intuition is a great way to activate and increase the strength of your third eye.

The final best way to exercise your third eye is to strengthen your psychic abilities. Whenever you experience one of the claims, allow yourself to fully embrace it. If it is showing you something or encouraging you to do something or trust a certain piece of information with no logical explanation, do your best to follow it. When you do, you will be strengthening the ability and your connection to your third eye.

Opening your third eye is a process. There is the process of opening it for the first time, and then the process of keeping it open. When you nurture your third eye, you will find that life is incredible and much simpler than you may have ever believed it could be. Our third eye can be considered our own built-in "northern star" guiding us in the direction we need to go. When we follow it and we listen to what it has to say, we are naturally guided to where we need to be in order to have the best experiences.

You have likely had many instances where you followed your third eye's guidance without knowing it since your third eye speaks to you through your intuition. When you open it intentionally, however, it becomes easier to follow and explore intentionally, and not go in a different direction because of any fear you may have of listening to your inner voice. When you are not intentionally listening to it and are unaware of the power of your third eye, it can be easy to be led astray and then end up feeling guilty or out of place because you did something you did not want to or that was not good for you despite something inside you telling you that you should have never done it in the first place.

When you are opening your third eye, ensure that you set aside time to continue doing it. There may be times where you don't always focus on it, but overall you should invest a few hours per week on working with your third eye chakra. This will help ensure that you are staying connected with it and that it is serving you in the most powerful way possible. As a result, you will find that life is much more balanced, fulfilling, satisfying, and purposeful. You will find more meaning in your life, and you will find that it is easier to follow your internal compass without fear that you are doing the wrong thing. In fact, you will have a much easier time being yourself, and the judgment and beliefs of others will not have such a strong ability to impact your own beliefs and you will be able to feel much freer.

# Chapter 3: Techniques to Awaken the Third Eye Chakra

## Activating and Maintaining the Third Eye Function

Specific mudras, or chants in the Hindu and Ayurvedic philosophies, are said to help activate and maintain the health of each chakra. For the Third Eye chakra it is recommended to chant "OM" in a quiet place for 1 – 20 minutes. There are also musical compositions that are designed to resonate with each specific chakra based on their individual tonal frequency. The frequencies for the Third Eye chakra are noted at 144 Hz, 288 Hz and 576 Hz.

Meditation is by far the most widely used practice for tapping into the Third Eye. While there are numerous forms of meditation, the basic idea is to slow down the thought process. How many times have we had the word for something on the tip of our tongue yet the more we try to think of what it is, the harder it is to recall? And later we find that when we have taken our minds off of it, the word comes to us easily and instantly!

This is why sleep stages and brain waves are inclusive, because many successful practitioners of meditation have described its purpose as bringing cognitive awareness to deeper levels of brain function where theta and delta waves are distinct. It is here where we are proposed to develop control over stress reduction and the healing processes of our bodies as seen naturally occurring in Stage IV sleep.

Dr. Nipun Aggarwal, MD, MBA, MHT, and José Silva are two notable authorities who have developed approaches to "mind control," training our mind's eye to consciously, effectively, and almost immediately regulate bodily functions for optimal health. These approaches are also geared toward maintaining focus and peace of mind in challenging and stressful, everyday situations, memorizing and quickly recalling vast amounts of information, as well as fluent problem solving beyond our five senses.

Using the third eye does not mean developing magical powers or becoming a psychic. It actually implies controlling your mind more effectively and enjoying a deeper sense of intuition to your surroundings. Unfortunately, this shift does not happen overnight, you will need to dedicate your life to spiritual practices that involves practicing awareness of the mind every day.

## The First Opening

Choose a day when you have lots of free time ahead of you, for instance at the start of a weekend. This lets you focus intimately on the eye-opening practices. Usually, it gets easier after the first opening. You can do it with friends or alone. It is preferable if you wear light-colored clothes. The first opening isn't very intense; you might just feel a tingling between the eyebrows.

- Technique

- Go to a quiet, tranquil place where you are sure not to be bothered for at least an hour.

- Light candles around the place

- Remove your shoes, watch, tie, belt and any other restrictive clothing or jewelry

- Lie down on the floor, carpet, blanket or mat with your arms on your sides and palms facing up

- Close your eyes, relax for about 3 minutes and them hum for 5 to 10 minutes

Phase 1

- Begin breathing through the throat gradually becoming aware of the vibration within the larynx

- Continue breathing for 5 to 10 minutes and in case your body or consciousness moves, let it be

Phase 2

- While maintaining the friction in the throat, shift your awareness to the region between your eyebrows

- It is important that you flow with your body's energy. Do not pay attention to time

Phase 3

- Place your palm on the area between the eyebrows about 3 to 5 centimeters away from the skin

Phase 4

- You can have the hand in phase 3 position or by your side

- With the eyes closed and larynx vibrating, begin to look for a vibration or tingling between the eyebrows.

- You may also feel a blurry pressure, density or weight

- Do not focus too hard, just remain vacant and let things take their own course

Phase 5

- As soon as you feel a vibration or something between your eyebrows try to connect it to the friction in your throat.

- The vibration will gradually become subtle yet more intense at the same time.

- Some people may feel the vibration in other parts of the body or on the entire forehead. This is normal; just focus on the vibration between the eyebrows.

Phase 6

- Stop the vibration in the Larynx

- Focus on the vibration between the eyebrows

- Be very still and try to focus on the energy around you

- Be aware of any light or colors between the eyebrows

Remember

- Keep your eyes closed throughout the process

- Do not grasp or focus too much on the region between the eyebrows as this might block the process

- If you are practicing with friends, do not touch each other

- If the experience overwhelms you, open your eyes to come back to normal consciousness

- For the first experience, the manifestations of the eye are not as important as getting the technique right. Minor bodily movements such as twitching as well as flashing in and out of consciousness may also occur during the first opening. Ignore them and perfect your technique as if nothing happened.

## Learning How To Meditate

To begin with, you will need to find the right environment. Choose a place where you can be left alone for at least 30 to 45 min and is relatively quiet. It doesn't need to be completely silent, but try finding a place where you will not be distracted a lot.

Start By Getting Into A Meditative Posture

Sitting on the ground with crossed legs, straight back and hands resting on the knees is considered to be a very effective meditative posture. If you're unable to sit on the ground, sit on a chair and keep your back straight. Support your upper body using your abdominal muscles, and do not allow your back to slouch over. Keep your shoulders down and point your chest out.

Relax Your Body

All of us hold tensions in our body while going through our daily life, which makes focusing very difficult. You will not realize how tensed your muscles are until you consciously try to relax them. Roll your head from side to side to loosen up your body, allow your neck muscles to release and your shoulders to drop.

## Relax Your Mind

This is one of the most essential parts of opening the third eye. Perhaps, it is also the most challenging one because you will need to remove all thoughts from your head. You can do this by focusing your attention on any one aspect of the physical world, whether it's the sensation of the ground under you, sound of traffic moving past or your breath going in and out.

While it's nearly impossible to eliminate all thoughts, if a thought does come into your mind, just acknowledge it and allow it to disappear from your mind. You will need a lot of patience and practice to clear your thoughts effectively. People generally find it very difficult to meditate during the first 10 to 20 min. Give yourself some time to transition from the world outside to a meditative state.

## Develop A Habit Of Meditating

The more you think about meditating, the better you'll get at it. You can think about meditation while eating your food, going for a walk or even while brushing your teeth. Even by meditating for just 5 min a day, you will train yourself to become more aware mindfully over time. Use a timer while meditating, as it will stop you from wondering how much time you've already spent meditating.

Open The Intuitive Part Of The Brain

Begin by observing the world around you. People who are generally shy tend to be more intuitive than the average person simply because they spend a lot of time observing other people; and by doing so they develop a higher understanding of things like facial expression, body language and other types of non-explicit communication. These people are very good at detecting sexual chemistry, lies, hidden messages and sarcasm.

You can practice intuition by going to a public place like a cafe, restaurant or park on your own and simply observe other people around you. Try to listen into their conversation without being overbearing or rude. Try to create a story in your mind on how these people got together or about what they are talking about or any other information that you find interesting. The more you will do this, the better you'll get at it.

You can also practice it while sitting around the table with your friends or family, try being quiet for some time and just listen to what they are talking about. Observe people who are not participating in the conversation and watch their reaction to the ongoing interaction. Try and imagine what they might be thinking about when they are not talking. The more you practice it, the better you'll get at.

Dreams Are Important

People with psychic powers generally believe that dreams can carry messages that can serve as a warning. To analyze your dreams start documenting them. The best way to do this is to maintain a dream diary kept next to your pillow. After you have documented a few dreams, try to find connections between them and check whether any part of your dreams has come true.

Try Following Your Gut Instinct

Have you ever felt peculiar about a place, event or person that you really can't put into words? Have you strongly felt that a certain situation might occur without having any evidence to back your feeling? These kinds of feelings are called gut instincts, and all of us have it in different degrees. Most people overlook their gut instincts and try to live their lives on the basis of rational thinking. Next time you have such a feeling, make a note of it and check if it actually comes true. Also try to determine if these feelings connect to your life in any way.

Always keep in mind that just because you have a gut feeling about something it doesn't really mean that it would come through. While it may come true, it could take months or even years for it to take place, which is why it will always help to make a note of these feelings so that when it happens you know for sure that you already knew about it.

## Experiences After The Opening Of The Third Eye

After your third eye opens you will go through some unusual experiences. While many of the experiences will be pleasant, there are some that might not be. If you feel some activity or pressure in the center of your forehead, it means that either your third eye has already opened or will open very soon.

Seeing Through The Third Eye

The Third Eye lets you to see past the visual images around you. With it, you can sense and visually interpret the energy around you. As you watch people walk in the park, you will grasp much more than just the abstract concept of random people walking in the park. You begin to see the interplay between the motion, energy, and intention in a vivid internal visual map. Life, therefore, becomes almost tangible to you.

While our physical eyes are blind to energy and can only see the results of energy, the Third Eye allows one to visualize where the energy is, to understand it and to actually see it. Our eyes are designed to see light while the third eye helps you process the energy you interact with in a precise manner.

Having an open Third Eye may seem like something mystical at first, but it merely is a new way that helps your mind communicate with the rest of your senses. This communication is direct and so uninhibited that you can accurately predict events and perceive potentials that are not physically present. This is a skill that is real that has been experienced by people from as early as the Paleolithic period.

## What To Expect After The Third Eye Has Opened

After your third eye has opened, do not be surprised when you go through some unusual experiences. This will have a lot to do with what you see. For example when you are very tired after a long day's work and are about to sleep, you might see different kinds of images in the eye of your mind after you close your physical eyes.

Many of these images won't make a lot of sense and will be blurred or vivid. There are a number of dimensions you can reach with an opened third eye and you will experience them gradually. It all depends on your thought's vibration levels. The higher your vibration levels the more dimensions you will be able to explore. If you're seeing blurred visions, you will need to further strengthen your spiritual powers. Reaching a higher state of meditation will help you see more clearly with your third eye.

### Higher And Lower Dimensions

If the vibrations of your thoughts are low then you will most likely see visions from a lower dimension. The lower dimension is the area where you will see restless souls. These are souls of the people who either killed themselves or could not forgive themselves for having done something in their lives. Since they are afraid of being judged they do not move into the higher dimension.

People who see visions from the lower dimension generally get scared of what they are seeing and regret opening their third eye. However, you don't have to remain in the lower dimension. Most people who remain at the lower dimension do so because the vibration created by their thoughts attracts this dimension. All you need to do is increase your vibration and step into a higher dimension.

If you would like to close your third eye, you can do so by avoiding spiritual practices, indulging in conversations that have nothing to do with the spiritual world and getting rid of every object in your surrounding that reminds you of it. While your third eye may not close immediately, slowly and gradually it will. However, it is important to note that once your third eye closes, it will take a lot of effort to open it back again.

With higher thought vibrations that include feelings of happiness, gratitude, love or peace you will be able to see more peaceful visions that would bring in a sense of fulfillment and relief to your soul. In this dimension, you will have visions of the hurt people go through and ideas that will help you make situations better along with feelings of compassion and forgiveness.

Sensitivity To Good And Bad Energies

Once your third eye has been awakened you'll become more sensitive to the energies of people around you. You will be able to detect between good and bad energies. It's always good to pick up good energies, because it will affect you positively. However, it is impossible not to pick up bad energies, which is why it's always good to avoid places where you know you will most likely to be hit by bad energies. This is one of the main reasons why people with stronger spiritual powers feel drained after spending time in a crowd, since they get hit by loads of bad energies.

When you're in the middle of bad energies try imagining being surrounded by positive energies in order to protect yourself. Think of something that makes you happy and continue to do so till you can get out of that atmosphere. It will stop your mind from being dragged into negative thoughts.

Once you're out of that situation and come back home, get under a shower with the water set to a slightly lower temperature than what you're used to. Imagine the water cleaning away all the bad energies that has affected you. As the water flows down from your body feel the bad energies flowing down with it. This is an excellent exercise to eliminate the effects of bad energy on your mind. As you do it for a couple of days, you will experience the cleansing effect more strongly. It will also help you become more focused and energetic throughout the day, and the ability of negative energies to disrupt your regular thought process will become weaker. It will also improve the quality of your life, your health, sleep, relationships and the general state of your mind.

Third Eye Opening Experiences

After your third eye has opened, during the initial period you might experience high-level vibrations that might scare you. The trick to get over this period is to stay calm and allow the vibrations to take control of your mind. As you stay calm, your mind will synchronize to the vibrations and will become accustomed to it.

You may see visions of beautiful places, which may include visions of a beautiful day or a beautiful house or anything that you feel is very peaceful and an enlightening place to be. Even though you will not be at such a place physically, your mind will reap all the benefits of being in such a place. The vastness of the images that you see in your vision will vary on the level of focus and meditation that you have achieved. While for some the visions might be in a frame wherein the mind will be aware of the darkness that's around the frame, for some the vision would be frameless and the clarity will be so great that the mind will no longer see any darkness or troubled images.

Closing the Third eye

Many people may choose to shut their third eye. The experiences post awakening and activation of the third eye can be quite overwhelming for them. In such cases, the easiest way to keep it shut is to not use it at all. Opening the eye requires effort and changes in your normal life. If you do mundane and meaningless things that don't require the use of the third eye, it remains closed by itself. Just keep yourself focused on the regular stream of things.

## THIRD EYE AWAKENING

For those who have opened their third eye, just push yourself back and become more grounded in the present. Keep bringing yourself to where you are and what is around you. Although you might start seeing and hearing more, you can control it. Just stop yourself from seeing or hearing the things you don't want to. It is as simple as closing your eyes when you don't want to watch something or skipping a channel on the television. Pay more attention to your physical presence and way of life. This will keep you grounded and prevent consciousness on higher levels. Don't drift your mind towards thoughts which are too deep and do not concern your daily life. All this helps to tone down the awareness of the third eye.

## Chapter 4: Guided Day Meditations to Awaken the Third Eye

If music is food for the soul, meditation is the most potent food for the third eye chakra. In fact, meditation is the best food for any endeavor in spiritual awakening. Meditation should be practiced alongside the exercises.

What Exactly is Meditation?

Meditation is a skill that can be learned and honed, just like any other skill we try our hand at. It does not require any special talents. On the other hand, it also needs to be approached without skepticism.

If you are new to meditation, you may feel a bit awkward and uncomfortable at first. However, the majority of people who experience the joys of meditation quickly learn to love it as a relaxing and enriching activity.

Meditation is basically an age-old practice established in ancient Indian traditions. It is practiced with the goal of opening the mind for deeper intuition and perception. There are also several very powerful meditations developed specifically to open the third eye and strengthen the pineal gland.

Meditation also helps you control your thoughts and your mind, putting you, as the proponents of Buddhism believe, in control of your life. This is an extremely empowering gift to have. So many things in life are out of our control—but by learning to control our thoughts, we can respond to situations wisely and calmly and make better choices. This skill becomes even more pronounced when your third eye chakra is awakened.

Meditation develops clarity and improves concentration and is possibly one of the best ways to relieve stress. These are just a few of the benefits of meditation. All of the physical and mental benefits—as well as the research that confirms them—are just too numerous to list here.

How does Meditation Work?

When you meditate, your brain enters into an alpha wavelength state, (which is different from the normal beta wavelength state that the brain resonates with). In this quiet and relaxed state, the mind becomes more open to receiving subtle messages and insights from our third eye. The regular practice of meditation allows you to enter more and more easily into the alpha wavelength state and over time, you can receive deeper wisdom, knowledge, and information from the non-physical realm. It also helps strengthen spiritual gifts.

Step 1: Choose a Location

For meditation to hit the primary target, you need to look for a place that there are minimal disturbances. A quiet place is all you need to start with. When you are choosing the site, you need to make sure that you will be consistent. The person to guide you on the meditation should be compatible with you. Your body, as well as the mind, needs to get used to the place that you will choose. A position that you will choose should be in charge of activating your third eye. That too you should consider when choosing the place.

Step 2: Choose the Time with an Intention

After you, through with the first step, work on the second step; that is, selecting the time that you will be going for the guided meditation sessions.

You will need to go for the sessions daily so that they can be useful. The time that you will decide to be having the sessions should be reasonable. You should remain fixed at the time that you will choose. Think of the time that will suit you best, and your body, as well as the mind, should be free and in a relaxation mood. You need to avoid scheduling the sessions immediately before or after the time that you take your meals. When you choose a morning, it will work best for you. But that does not mean that any other time is not appropriate. All that is needed when you choose any additional time besides morning is you maintain consistency.

## Step 3: Make Some Stretches Before You Begin the Meditation Session

You need to make some stretches before you go to the meeting since you will have to sit longer in the room. You can have a more comfortable time as you meditate on how to open your third eye so that you can realize the power that is in you. When you do this any time before getting into the meditation sessions, you will go to a deeper length of your mental framework. You can try bending over as you try to touch the toes for at least a minute. You can stretch your arms above the head as a way of relaxing. Do not forget to lay on your back and make sure that your feet are in the air at ninety degrees with the body.

Step 4: Position Yourself

Meditation cannot take place while you are standing. You need to adopt a sitting position where you feel relaxed, and you need to cross your legs. If you find this posture disturbing and not comfortable, decide to change and take one which is not difficult for you. A position that will make you relax and focus quickly on your breathing, as well as meditation, is what you need to consider. You should sit on the floor while you close your legs so that you will meditate better on how to open your third eye and access to the hidden spiritual treasures. Your chest should be open and your back straight. Consider placing your hands either on the knees or the lap depending on the position that you will better. Your head needs to be upright and close the eyes gently so that you can get into the world of meditation.

## Step 5: Relax

After you adopt a posture that you feel comfortable in, the next logical thing that you need to do is give your body the chance to settle. Meditation cannot take place when you are not relaxed. Be mindful of how your body is feeling and if there are feelings that you need to work on them before the actual meditation, do that. Make sure that your entire body is relaxed and ready to begin the session. Pay attention to all parts of the body each at a time as you sit as well as relax. Shift your mind from any worry that you may be having and be ready to pay attention to the present moment. As you breathe in and out, make sure you are feeling your body expanding and contracting when you take every breath.

## Step 6: Breath

Breathing is a crucial technique in meditation. Be focused on how you breathe in and out and put your full attention on how you are breathing. Take deep breaths from time to time on the count of three as you inhale and exhale.

Step 7: Empty the Mind

At this point, you will begin focusing on the third eye, which is at the center of the forehead. With still, your eyes are closed, move your eyes on the direction of the third eye. Throughout the entire meditation process, you need to maintain the focus without moving the eyes from that position. Remaining on the emphasis, count from one hundred moving backwards but do not worry if you are not able to experience the third eye at that moment. You can take quite some time to get used to the process of meditation. It can even take longer to activate your third eye, but that should not worry you. All you need to do is maintain consistency, and with time all things shall work out.

Step 8: Access the Third Eye

When you are through with counting from a hundred backward, it is time that you try to access the sight. Make sure that you had maintained the focus in the previous steps so that this point will be a success. When you have the attention, you will notice that all things are dark apart from your third eye. When the eye is active, your brain will be as well relaxed and functioning on an entirely new level. All the sides of the brain will work in unison, and you will feel the energy that surrounds you. You will feel a new energy level running through your body as well as around you. That is the moment you will know that you got access to your third eye. When you focus on an object or image strongly, that is the time that you know that you are accessing the eye. Your mind needs to be consumed by the object or image fully for that to happen.

## Step 9: Work on Experiencing Your Third Eye

Everyone has a different way of reacting to the activation of their third eye. You may experience your mind flashing visual effects and any other experiences and scenes that you may have come through. It can be a way of seeing your thoughts like the way they appear if they can be laid out. As you continue focusing on experiencing your third eye, you will work on opening the eye slowly by slowly.

Step 10: Maintain Your Focus on the Third Eye

You need to remain focused on the third eye for about ten to fifteen minutes. You may have a headache during the very first sessions but know that it is a normal thing that will happen to almost every beginner. There is no need to get worried since the headache will be no more as you get used to the practice. You have to train yourself to fully appreciate your third eye and try to maintain your focus on one image. Amongst the pictures that will appear in your mind, pay attention to one that you decide to choose. Make sure you work to keep the mind centered on the focus that you have made. When you maintain your focus on the third eye, you will find it open slowly. That will mean that you had achieved what your aim was when you were deciding to go meditation. Your third eye will open, and you will have a great experience with the precious gift that is in you.

Step 11: Get out Meditation Slowly

When you finally achieve what you intended, the next thing to do is bring yourself out of the meditation. Remove your focus from your third eye slowly still maintain the relaxation mood that you were in when in the whole process. Your guide will let you know that you have to be aware of your breath. You can choose to count as a way to still focus on your breathing when working on bringing your mind from the meditation. Open your eyes slowly to end the entire process finally.

In cases when you need to open your third eye any other time, practice the above steps, and it will be easier this time around. That is because it will not be the first time to do that. Work on making your body feel better as well as become in touch with the inner self. However, that will not come immediately, since you need to practice the meditation process, and it will make you go to greater heights. You will be more in touch with yourself as well as the energy in you and around you. That is the main idea of meditating to open your third eye.

There are signs that you will experience to show that your eye is open. Once you manage to open the third eye, you will no longer have self-doubt. You will have a desire to research as well as learn more. You will be more sensitive to spirits, and you may see them from time to time. You will be wiser and will learn from your past mistakes. The chances are that you will be more creative, and you will feel divine inspirations more often. You will achieve great potential, and you will have joy and experience a healthy life once you can connect with the spirits. You will find the world a place of harmony to live in, and you will appreciate your life more. When you finish the self-journey, do not be mean but work to show other buddies with a similar gift with you the way of self-realization.

## Chapter 5: The Powers of an Open Third Eye

### Freedom from Anxiety, Stress, and Worries

With every meditation session, your consciousness level increases. You will start achieving higher states of consciousness. The light inside you illuminates you. It takes away your insecurities and fears. Our worries are a product of our worldly burdens. With every step we take in our lives, the Karma has its effect. It keeps on piling up. We fail to recognize the impact of Karma and keep fretting over the results. Meditation gives us the power to ponder upon our actions and the resultant Karma. It all starts making sense and you can make amends. Clear thoughts give birth to reasoning. We also start giving weight to cause and not just the results. This helps in balancing the effect of Karma.

The illumination also makes you realize the importance of various things in life. You can prioritize things better. We do many things without setting up clear priorities. This creates a lot of backlash in form of pending mortgage, student loan, or unpaid credit card bills. These keep haunting our thoughts. Once you can see clearly inside yourself, you start understanding that most of the actions were unnecessary. You can also get out of them once you reason and align them properly. This is the best way to come clear from this vicious cycle of debts and liabilities.

☐ Victory Over Emotions

One of the biggest reasons for our distress is our emotions. Love, hatred, dislike, and affection are some of the free-flowing emotions. We attach undue importance to things. The negative energies and emotions accumulate and make us sad. Most of these emotions and energies are avoidable. When you look deep inside yourself, you find that most of your outbursts were unreasonable and uncalled for. You could have avoided the negative energies by suppressing them. These eventually lead to sadness. Your inner light will give you the wisdom to introspect. This time is entirely yours. In this moment, you are unchallenged. There is no victory or loss. You are in complete control. There is no ego or tussle. You take rational decisions. This leads to the birth of positive decisions. You are able to shun negative energies. It is relieving and light. You become happy from within. You get mature and become affable in real terms. You are able to take proactive steps towards improving your health and relationships. You can make prudent decisions towards strengthening your career and financial situation. The intuitive power of the third eye will help you in assessing your future course of action.

☐ You Start Changing from Within

Now, we know that meditation helps you in self-introspection. You understand the impact of Karma. You also understand the impact even the small steps would have on your life. You are able to predict the consequences of those actions. This knowledge helps in shaping up a new you. You become a better and improved human being. Your thought process starts changing from the root. Your worries and insecurities vanish slowly and gradually. This makes you more confident and strong. As your Third eye opens up your physical, emotional and mental well being improves. This starts reflecting in your overall personality. You mellow down. You become calm yet confident.

Your path to success becomes clear. Your goals become clear and the path leading up to them also gets crystal clear. There is no confusion. The mind makes it way through the darkness. It is no more just an entangled structure of nerve cells. It gets illuminated.

You start realizing the power of your mind. It is a powerhouse. It gets illuminated and you know the things in place. Once the light comes the path gets clear. The challenge lies in bringing the light. The pineal gland or the Ajna chakra needs to be illuminated and activated. This requires focus, dedication, and discipline. You will have to work your way till here with meditation. You will have to open your Third eye inwards. This will need patience and determination. It is a doable task. You will just have to dedicate yourself to it. The path is not tough. It only requires you to keep walking on it. The journey is calming and rewarding. You only need to take the first step towards it. It will lead you from there.

## It is Possible for Anyone to Activate the Third Eye Chakra

One of the most important things to understand in this whole process is that the third eye is in every person irrespective of their religion, race, or creed. Activating your third eye is a spiritual process and not a religious one. You can belong to any religion or faith and still practice it. It is not a worship of any god. It is self-realization. It is empowering yourself. It is all about knowing yourself inside-out. It is achieved through the process of meditation.

Most of us keep looking for information about ourselves outside. We ask for opinions about ourselves. We worry about the things people say about us. We care for those things. This leads to miseries. The opinions expressed by anyone are laced with prejudice and aided with a different perspective. They can never be unbiased or neutral. You have very little or nothing to gain from such opinions and everything to lose. You may start correcting yourself irrespective of the fact that you were never wrong in the first place. This would be counterproductive. But, still, this happens all the time in our lives. We start shaping ourselves into different people and not the way we want ourselves to be. You are trying to be an image of someone else. God created you in his image. Why would you want to be an image created by another mere mortal?

An illuminated third eye guides you to the path of self-correction based on rationality. The light shows you the right path. But, you need to bring this light. You need to open the third eye. You need to decalcify the pineal gland or activate the Ajna chakra. With guided meditation and focus, it is possible for anyone to activate the third eye chakra and see the light. It is like awakening to a new consciousness. It cannot be corrupted in any manner because it comes from inside you. It is free of all blemishes.

The third eye chakra rests in your pineal gland. It is in the middle of the brain. It is the 'anchor of the soul'. It regulates your sleep cycles, sexual maturation, and vital hormones. It gets calcified with impurities over the time. The third eye meditation helps in decalcification of the pineal gland. It opens your mind.

### Eight Tips for Effective Energy Meditation

Whether you are doing energy meditation as core energy qigong, pranayama, meditation for a while, kundalini, or another method, or if you have just started, the follow these eight tips will help you advance. Many of these tips can also be applied to any other type of meditation.

Meditation is an activity that, for some time, concentrates your focus on a specific object or in a particular way. Energy meditation means that you use creativity and the sense of Life's energy, prana, or "qi" as your focus. The energy centers and pathways in your body are a great way to meditate because they are an effective way to follow your mind. It's fun and usually feels good as you grow your skills.

Energy meditation motivates you in your body at this stage, which is an effective way to "get out of your head." It also has some benefits for your health, including activating your natural response to relaxation, better posture, tension release, better circulation, deeper breathing, coherent brain and heart function, and improved immune response. Energy therapy helps you feel relaxed, optimistic, and vital. It brings you, more importantly, to the core level of "whom you are" and "what you are to do." It ties you to your internal direction, deeper meaning, and connection to Life.

We concentrate on the Chinese qigong method and Core Energy Meditation on three primary energy centers ("dahntee-ens") inside your body:

1. Your lower dantian or body core in your lower abdomen that is connected to your inner vitality.

2. Your central dantian or heart center in your chest which deals with your refined senses and

qualities of interaction with others, including appreciation, gratitude, confidence, compassion, and love.

3. Your upper dantian or Mind center in the center of your brain, which relates to your intuition, mental powers, insight, concentration, and ability to watch your experiences calmly without being overwhelmed.

You may not imagine or feel much when you first practice imagining and feeling your energy centers. It might be a obstacle to keep the training based on them. It is also common to contact one, but not the other or two and not the third. Your experience depends on your natural vision and kinesthetic sensing capacity, the degree to which your energy centers are triggered, and how much you have experienced inside your body.

Wherever you are in the ability to imagine and feel inside your mind, it's all right. You can benefit from the practice, regardless of your current skills. When you practice consistently over time, you will slowly be able to perceive, observe, absorb, distribute, develop, and maintain your internal life force.

You will also notice positive effects as you increase your ability to feel inner guidance, to make good choices, to be present, and to follow your best intentions. You come to feel better in your body, heart, mind, and spirit, healthy and positive. You will establish a consistently reliable, optimistic, clear, and coherent private, energetic vibration, or what I would like to call a "core energy state."

Eight Efficient Energy Meditation Tips: 1. Practice daily, first, and foremost. If you only exercise if you feel that you need it, remember that in practice, you have much more to do than use it to relax and go to the core when you "stress" (which is undoubtedly important). If you practice each day, your experience and tensions during the last 24 hours will be better handled so that you approach Life in a much more transparent, more relaxed, positive, and focused way.

You can also note the difference when you miss a day's workout when unresolved stress clouds your perception and affects your feeling. In the first few years of practice, it is common to experience the release of "old things," which can bubble into your consciousness as you meditate. The more tensions you release from the past, the freer you can live in the present.

To encourage your daily exercises, I recommend you choose a time that is appropriate for you, maybe 15-20 minutes, and plan it every day at the same time (for example, in the early morning). Even if it is challenging to wake up early, you are probably starting to look forward to waking up and joining a "core energy state." The main reason for daily practice is that each time you sit down, you can move into practice and build on what you did the day before. You're going to stay in the flow. If you practice sporadically or seldom, you will "always begin." 2. 2. If you have exercised regularly for some time, you may want to consider increasing the time you spend on your practice. While 15-20 minutes per day is good, meditating longer is likely to intensify and strengthen benefits. The longer you meditate, the deeper, clearer, and quieter you can enter.

For the first 10-15 minutes of practice, a lot of mental chat is healthy, which slows down slowly the longer you continue. When you sit for 30-40 minutes or longer, you may be in a quieter state for more time. The extra time will increase the effect in your mind and body and make this a more accurate point of reference to which you can return more quickly.

For increasing your time, you can find one more extended session a week or two longer sessions a week on weekends. But don't give yourself too much to make it a mission. Lengthen your time with the increase of your natural desire.

3. In addition to increasing the total time, you can increase the time you spend working on any energy center. For example, you can comfortably concentrate on your brain core, but you will find it harder to focus on your heart or lower abdomen. One or more of these centers are commonly more easily focused on, and one or more are more challenging.

You may want to spend more time at the energy centers that you are most familiar with when you first start training. That's okay, to build your confidence. However, as you start, your training and your Life will be most advanced when you spend extra time focusing on the energy centers you think least or are most challenged. These are probably the places where your flow of energy is not as fluid and free. You may store long-lasting feelings or traumas in these places.

Spend more time on these areas with a positive mind, a sense of understanding of how your body works to keep you safe, and relaxed analytical focus will start releasing these kept pressures so that your energy system performs more entirely and becomes more deeply integrated. One way to do this is to turn your attention to a sense of spacious quiet in the center of every energy center. Just being in an energy center can have a therapeutic effect, if you sit there without attempting to do anything or make anything happen.

In the Daoist tradition, it is seen as healthy when you begin your practice to focus more on your lower dantian or lower abdominal energy core. When your energy builds up in this center, your energy naturally will flow up to the middle dan tian or heart center, then up to the upper dan tian or mind center. Whether you pursue the progress or another method depending on your specific needs, it's a good idea to start and finish your research by collecting energy from your lower dan tian.

4. To support your lower dantian's strong vitality well for your body. Excess energy is necessary to focus your attention strongly and expand your

practice. Your physical health is the source of this extra energy. Track these five things to improve your physical vitality:

- Go with your "To-Do List,"

- Get enough rest,

- Consume a variety of foods as fresh and as close as possible to their natural state,

- Drink enough water to remain well-hydrated (most of us have around 64 ounces a day) and

- Exercise periodically If you have committed themselves to practice early, didn't eat quality food, but are wary of your life and haven't gone to bed soon enough, didn't get well hydrated and haven't exercised properly, you probably won't have the energy to have a good practice. You can devote a lot of time to the opening, triggering, clearing, and integration of your energy centers with enough physical vitality.

5. Imagine and feel breathing through any energy center to activate and clear it. As you inhale,

imagine and think that you fill your breath with that energy center. When you exhale, imagine and feel that you empty that power center and release any tension. Try to believe that your breath brings light and space into your energy center when you inhale. Try to imagine that you have any congestion or density when you exhale.

This technique can also be used to pressure anywhere in the body. Consider and sound like you breathe into the area around the narrow area, softening the edges. Draw your breath directly into the center of the space where you feel stress or density. Imagine and feel like your breath brings light, openness, and space into that area. Exhale any density or density.

6. You can also spend more time on the links between the energy centers. Three donations are linked to the Central Channel or the Middle Mai Channel. This stream is noticeable and feels like a vertical pipe running from your perineum to the middle of your body (in front of the spine, but also the tail) at the top of your head. This channel binds and combines the three dantians into a cohesive balanced system.

You might feel that one energy center is reliable, open, transparent, and others are dull, tense, or cloudy. Through the Central Channel, you can imagine and feel the connection between them as a way to activate and clear the nude center. You can also visualize and sense the breath moving through the two as you breathe in and out.

Another explanation is that you feel open in the energy centers, but lack a sense of integration. You may feel they're not aligned vertically, or they don't work well together. For instance, your mind doesn't work with your heart and body. They are not in harmony. We are not in sync. Your mind thinks something, your heart feels something else, and your body wants something entirely different.

If this is the case, the Central Channel can be perceived and felt like a bright, vertical column with the three Dantians in its center and breathing through this channel. During my training, I like to do this at several stages to refresh my focus. I also complete my practice by inhaling the central channel and breathing down the primary chain several times. Then, before I open my eyes, I collect energy in the lower dan tian.

The bottom line of energy therapy is that it is person-specific. You start by learning good ways. Once you master the forms, you can adapt them to your particular needs and what happens to you at any time. The more you understand the practice and the more sensitive you are to your internal flow or fluidity, the more you know how to proceed. Energy meditation makes you aware of your inner direction.

7. After you have practiced a method or form of meditation extensively through a guided video, you can try to practice yourself without the audio. After months or years of training, this could be. Offer your inner guidance to refine and grow your inner strength. Take time to open areas of pressure, use your breathing, and allow your conscious presence in your energy field to lead the way.

Whenever your mind wanders, notice and embrace it and return gently, as you stay present, accept anything, and return to let energy flow smoothly through you, I believe you are going to discover more profound confidence in your more profound life force.

This brings us to the 8th tip for adequate exercise.

8. You have a firm and clear intention for your practice when you sit to meditate. Having a strong "why" leads to an unwavering focus. For example, in meditation, my purpose is to become a clear channel through which life energy can flow. I call this a state of core energy. I feel free, calm, purposeful, clear, and whole in such a state. When I move into life from this state, I can feel and follow what I am to do at every moment, my service to others. When I sit down in my mind to meditate profoundly and, my practice has more energy.

Remember why you are meditating and sharing your intention when you sit down to practice. See whether this helps to motivate you and strengthen your focus. I hope that the eight guidelines above will help to cultivate your meditative experience, refine the energy of your life, and enhance the positive feelings of vitality and purpose.

### Benefits of Opening Your Third Eye

Here are a lot of benefits from the decalcification or activation of your third eye or also called your pineal gland. I see a lot of people are wondering how to know their third eye is opened or decalcified.

Our everyday life leads to calcification of the third eye and therefore, it doesn't work at its full potential by producing DMT and connecting us to other worlds.

If you have successfully decalcified and activated your third eye, you should observe a lot of benefits.

I have listed some of the most popular benefits of third eye activation.

Benefits of opening your third eye.

A lot of people believe that the third eye functions as a spiritual gateway through which you can see beyond time and space. In short, activating the third eye, your perceptions exceed the limits of the material, physical word and the mind awakens and connects you to levels of being where time doesn't exist. And this leads to a number of great advantages:

1. Greater awareness / Awakening.

Advantages of awakening your third eye.Awakening your third eye metaphysically opens our eyes from a deep spiritual lethargy.

This allows us to begin to perceive the "truth" that surrounds us.

What this means is that you will begin to see the world we live in is full of control and inequality and is not in harmony with the rest of the Universe.

You will feel a desire to be free and live in a world filled with love, compassion and truth. Eventually, you will feel and see the interconnectedness with everything around you in nature and will feel a deep connection with the Universe.

This is a deep sense that allows you to see the beauty in all things and to realize that your physical I is not your true nature.

2. Psychic Powers / Empathy.

Your instincts are as a well-adjusted compass that points you in the "right" direction to achieve what your soul is looking for.

It's almost like you know what will happen and what will be the results of certain events. That's why some people think that the most notable prophets of our time had their third eye opened.

The feeling that we are all part of the same whole also becomes clear and you are capable of empathy with others, knowing that they are part of the same universal consciousness.

3. Laws of attraction / Space order.

Opening your third eye chakra. As a result of the opened third eye, the third eye chakra is activated, which in turn will help to balance your chakra system.

When you are energized and in harmony with the Universe, you are like a giant magnet for events, people, situations etc. By harnessing the power of the positive intent, gratitude and love, you can manifest much more beauty in your life. You will notice that the number of useful "coincidences" will be greatly increased.

4. Vivid dreams / Lucid dreaming.

This means that you will feel that you can control your dreams and you will be able to realize your true infinite self and the infinite possibilities that exist in a state of sleep.

Additionally, you will realize that this world of dreams is the same as the "real world" in which we live, for example the fact that we have unlimited possibilities and we are all masters of our own universe.

5. Astral travel / Astral projection.

When the third eye connects to this level of existence where there is no time and space, our soul is able to rise above the physical body and astral travel in time and space.

Astral projection is one of the benefits coming with the activation of your third eye.It has the ability to go anywhere in the universe and at any time in the universe.

Many people belive that when we dream, we actually astral travel, and with fully opened third eye we are able to astral travel while we are awake, for example, when we meditate.

6. Imagination / Creativity.

With activated pineal gland, you are continuously connected to the plane of existence where our souls reside.

In the plane of existence, there is no time or space, just an endless love and truth – everything that has happened and will ever happen already exists in the plane of existence.

After connecting to it, you will find that your imagination and creativity are super charged and you are able to find solutions to problems easier because all the solutions to all problems already exist in this place. Along with the ability to have vivid dreams and lucid dreaming, this will spark your imagination to a whole new level.

## Chapter 6: Psychic Abilities

What Are Psychic Abilities?

Psychic abilities are another interesting topic in spirituality. It should be noted that when you practice the exercises in this book, especially the meditation techniques, then you will definitely awaken your psychic abilities. This is because there is really nothing supernatural about psychic abilities, especially when your chakras are strong and healthy. There are many kinds of psychic abilities. Let us discuss them one by one:

Clairvoyance

Among the different psychic abilities out there, the psychic ability of clairvoyance is probably the most common. Once again, clairvoyance is the ability of clear-seeing. But, just to give you another effective exercise that you can do, here is something that you can try:

Assume a meditative posture and relax. Think of a place in your house. Make it specific, for example, your bathroom or the other room in your house. Now, visualize it as clearly as you can. Pay attention to small details such as the arrangement of objects, the floor, ceiling, walls, and others.

Take note of what you see. Now, open your eyes, and check if you were able to "see" the said room in your mind's eye.

This is an excellent exercise that will allow you to travel and see places only with the power of clairvoyance. For this exercise, you can also use the visualization screen that we have talked about. Do not rush in doing this technique. Take as much time as you need to take note of the details in your mind's eye.

Now, in your first several attempts, you will most likely fail to see everything clearly and correctly, but do not allow this to discourage you. Instead, just maintain a positive mindset and keep on practicing. Do not allow failures to discourage you. You will never truly fail as long as you keep on trying. The more that you practice this technique, the more that you will get good at it. This is simply how it is when you try to learn a psychic ability. It is just like learning any other new skill. So, just keep on practicing and doing your best. After some time, as long as you are patient enough, you will soon notice some progress. You will start to see that you are more able to envision the place in your mind more clearly and that you can tell correctly where certain things are as if you were actually in the place that is being visualized. All these use the power of the third eye. If you train yourself well, then this will allow you to see different places and dimensions. Although this may seem like a simple visualization exercise, it is also very effective. In fact, if you come to think about it. All of these spiritual practices are actually very simple, but it just a matter of practicing it sincerely and continuously that can create a big difference.

Pyrokinesis

Pyrokinesis is the psychic ability to control fire. Yes, there are some people who can do this. Unfortunately, there are many scammers and hacks out there that use trickery to do a similar act. The truth is that pyrokinesis is real, and you can control fire with your mind. Here is an exercise that will allow you to do this. For this exercise, you will need to use some matches:

Assume a meditative posture and relax. Now, light a match and focus on the flame. You should try to connect to this flame and make it "jump" out of the matchstick. There is no right or wrong way to do this. You have to find your own way. The key is simply to focus on the flame and then be one with it. Once you are with it, you will feel as if the flame has become an extension of yourself. This is the time when you can actually control the flame as if it were your arm or finger as if it were just another part of your body. You can now make it jump or move it to be separated from the matchstick.

This technique may take some practice. If you are just starting out, you might find it a challenge. In fact, out of 20 tried, you might only be able to do it once or even none at all. However, do not be discouraged and just keep on practicing. The more that you practice, the more that you will get good at it. This is just the first basic exercise for learning pyrokinesis. Once you get good at it, you can now try another exercise where you get to control the flame and make it dance; hence it is called as the dancing flame exercise. For this exercise, you will need a candle:

Assume a meditative posture and relax. Light a candle in front of you and just focus on the flame. Be one with the candle flame. The more that you focus on the candle, the more that you will feel as if you were being one with it. Try to associate yourself with the candle or at least make it as an extension of yourself. The key here is to focus on the candle flame and not to allow other thoughts to exist in your mind. Now, once you feel like you are attuned with the flame, will it to bend to the right (or to any direction of your choice), and then make it bend toward another direction, and so on. You might want chant, "Bend to the right (or any direction of your choice)," to impress your will upon it. Another technique is to visualize the candle flame bending or leaning in the direction where you want it to bend. Now, if you get good at this, then you can take it a step further. This time, what you need to do is to make the flame move so that it separates from the wick. This is the same as the first exercise with the match. This is the way to extinguish the flame. Another technique is to visualize the flame getting smaller and smaller until it finally disappears.

Now, the next part is probably the hardest part. This technique is a way to light up a candle. The steps are as follows:

Visualize the molecules of the candle. See the molecules moving faster and faster as they heat up. As you do this, see and feel the wick of the candle getting red and hotter and hotter. Continue with this visualization. Believe in it and in its power. Soon enough, with enough willpower, the candle will light up.

This is an advanced technique so do not expect to be able to do it easily. You might want to practice these techniques as a routine. First, try to just move or make the candle flame bend, and then have it separated from the wick to snuff it out, and then finally relight it back. Once you can do all these, you can easily use the fire element in anything. This is how spiritual masters can set an object in fire from a distance. Indeed, this is also not easy to master. But, if you feel like you are attuned to the element of fire, then this is probably the psychic ability that is best for you.

Telekinesis

Telekinesis, or simply TK, is another famous psychic ability. It refers to the ability to move, or influence injects with the mind. Now, it should be noted that telekinesis is divided into two kinds: micro telekinesis and macro telekinesis. Micro TK refers to the ability to influence randomness or odds. For example, being able to influence a random number generator or a shuffled deck of cards. Macro TK refers to how most people understand what TK is, which is the moving of objects with the mind. For you to better understand micro and macro TK, it is best to do so using an actual practice:

Micro TK

For this exercise, all you need is a coin. Remember that micro TK is about influencing the outcome of randomness or odds. Here, you will use your mind to influence the outcome of a coin flip. The first step is to get a coin – any coin will do as long as it is well balanced, which means that when you flip it, it will randomly be a head or a tail side. The weight should be distributed equally on both sides. Do not worry; it seems that all ordinary coins are like this, so just use your regular coin. The second step is to choose your side: head or tail side. What you will do is to influence your chosen side so that it will come up with every toss or flip of the coin. Finally, you have to influence the said coin as you flip it 100 times.

Now, in theory, when you flip a coin 100 times, then the final outcome should be 50 heads and 50 tails, or somewhere close to it. But, if you can apply micro TK, then it should show a significant difference, like 70 head side and 30 tail side, if head is your chosen side.

So, how exactly do you do this? How should you apply micro TK? Well, the best way to do it is with your mind, and that is by using your will and visualization. The steps are as follows:

Relax. Telekinesis is more effective when you are relaxed. Realize that you are not forcing something to happen. Rather, you are making or letting it happen. Now, let us assume that your chosen side is the head side. As you flip or toss the coin, visualize in your mind that it falls with head side up. As you do this, exercise a strong will, as if commanding the coin to do as you will.

Here is another technique that you can use:

Hold the coin in your hand. Now, just stare at it and focus on it. Be one with it as you try to be one with the flame. Just focus on it until it feels as if it has become a part of you. Now, once you feel that you are in control of it. Just use your willpower to influence it and make it give you the outcome that you want. As you flip the coin, feel that the coin is a part of you and just make it land the way you want it.

There is really no secret to this technique. It is all about becoming one with the coin and controlling it to make it do your will. Do not identify the coin as a separate object. Rather, you ought to feel as if you were the coin or that it is at least a part of you, like your arm or elbow. Be one with the coin. You are the coin.

This is just an example of how micro TK can be used. If you reach a point where it becomes easy for you to control the outcome of a coin flip, you can try other things, such as a shuffled deck of cards or a dice. If you are using a shuffled deck of cards, an exercise that you can try is to force a color. For example, think of a color (red or black) as you shuffle the deck of cards. The top card of the shuffled deck of cards should be the chosen color. Feel free to device your own way to practice micro TK. Once you acquire and develop this ability, you can use it for many purposes. In fact, there are those who claim that this can be used to influence the odds in the casino or even the lottery. You might be surprised, but there are real-life lottery winners who are psychics and spiritual practitioners. Take note, however, that psychic abilities are not really meant to make you rich. Instead, you should use them to help other people and grow more spiritually. Never lose the real purpose for practicing these things, and always cling to what is good.

Macro TK

Macro TK is exactly what most people understand when they encounter the word, telekinesis, and this is actually moving objects with your mind, such as moving a coin, ring, or even heavy objects like a television or a car. You might be wondering, is this really possible? Well, this might surprise you, but the answer is a resounding yes. You see, there is no limit to the power of your mind except the one that you have made against it. The following exercise will help you practice and experience macro TK:

Place a light object in a table in front of you. Now, focus on this object. Be one with it. Focus on it to such an extent that you see nothing but the object. Create a tunnel in your mind that connects you to the object and let nothing else exist but this. Feel and be one with the object. Now, in your mind's eye, see your astral hand reaching out and pushing the said object.

Did it move? Another way to do this is to simply use your willpower and just be one with the object as you make it move with your will. Now, most people may require the use of visualization. You can try both ways and see which one works best for you. Again, do not be discouraged if nothing happens on your first few attempts. Just keep on practicing.

Here is another exercise that you might want to try. This can help you to levitate something, which is also a part of macro TK. The steps are as follows:

Place a light object, preferably a feather, on your hands. Keep your hands in front of you with the palms facing upward. Feel the object resting on your palms. Feel how light it is. Now, we will use energy to levitate this object, and we will draw energy by using this chant: light as air, light as a feather. Keep chanting it for a few minutes as you connect to the object and will it levitate.

Instead of using a feather, you can also use aluminum foil. The aluminum foil might not levitate, but it will most probably move on your hand.

Take note that telekinesis, especially macro TK is considered an advanced psychic ability, so do not expect to be able to do these exercises immediately without spending enough practice. Still, this ability is something that is worth learning. Once again, do not allow it to make you lose your sight on what is truly important in your spiritual life. Remember that although acquiring psychic powers can be nice and interesting, it is not the end of spirituality.

Hydrokinesis

Hydrokinesis refers to the ability to control water. You might see some videos on this on YouTube. Unfortunately, many of those people who promote themselves on such sites are only looking for attention and their abilities seem sketchy or fake. So, the best way is still for you to try it out yourself. For this exercise, you will need a basin and a needle. The steps are as follows:

Fill the basin with water. Now, place the needle in the basin and let it float. Take note that hydrokinesis deals with water so you would want to focus on the water. The needle is only there to show you if what you are doing is working. Now, visualize pushing the water with your energy. You might want to mimic the action with your hand as if you were pushing it with your hand, although you are actually doing so only with the power of your mind. Push the water to one side. The needle should respond and be pushed towards that side/corner. Focus on the water. Be one with it and push it. You can also visualize a wave in the water and use that wave to move the water. Just realized all throughout and connect with the element of water.

Once you get good at this, you can take it a step further. Go to the sea or any body of water. Now, use your ability to manipulate the water. It is believed that once you master this technique, you can do wonders such as changing the course of a river or of the typhoon. You can actually be able to control water and direct its flow. However, just like any other interesting psychic ability, this also requires practice.

Clairsentience

Clairsentience, also known as clear-eyed information, is the ability to feel the subtle energy. If clairvoyance is more about the sense of sight, then clairsentience deals with feelings. This is not as hard as you might think. In fact, you probably have a good sense of clairsentience, and you are simply not aware of it. A common example of this is having a bad feeling and then something undesirable happens, such as an accident. Or, you might feel a positive energy only to realize that an angel just passed by. This is more about feeling, not just energy but also the quality of energy. So, how do you develop or practice this ability? Well, just keep on feeling energy. The best way to do this is to develop your empathic ability. You can use this exercise:

Make sure that you are in a public place, or anywhere where there are people around you. Now, look around you and try to find someone whom you feel is a nice person. You do not have to be logical about this, but let your intuition decide for you. Now, just focus discreetly on this person. Feel your heart chakra. Remember that your heart chakra is the center of emotions and universal love and oneness. Now, see and feel a ray of light shoot off from your heart chakra and let it connect with the heart chakra of the chosen person. This will serve as your link and connection to the person. The next step is to simply clear your mind. You should be able to receive impressions or thought and ideas, even emotions, from the person.

You are not limited to feeling only the energy of people, but you can also use your ability to sense the energy of a place. If you do not like to travel, you can even conjure the place in your mind's eye and try to feel it from there. Once again, just like the other skills, this one also takes practice. The key here is to get used to using your feelings to sense the subtle energy around you. The more that you practice this, the more sensitive you will be to the subtle energy.

Divination

The practice of divination is very common to those who are into spirituality. A common tool that is used by dowsers is the tarot cards. Now, this book will not define every tarot card as that can be a lot. Instead, you will learn how to use any kind of tarot decks. The way to do this is by using your intuition. So, how do you do this? Well, the truth is that all tarot cards communicate a message that you can decipher. Instead of giving each card a meaning that the manufacturer has provided, you can also come up with your own personal meaning. The way to do this is by using your intuition.

Now, there are no hard and fast rules on how to do this. You will want to pick a card or make a spread. Once you have the cards that you need to interpret, just relax and clear your mind and allow your intuition to take full reign. Look at the card and focus on it. How does it make you feel? Do you sense any ideas or emotions being evoked by the card? Take as much time as you can to understand the card. With enough practice, you will get good at this and be able to read any tarot cards. You should realize that tarot cards are just tools. They do not form rules or regulations. Instead, you use them to communicate to you a message. It would be impractical to memorize all the meanings of all the tarot cards, especially now that there are countless tarot cards out there.

Another method of divination is by using a pendulum. In this case, you will have to learn the art known as dowsing. Okay, what is a pendulum? A pendulum refers to any object that is suspended on a string or chain. Before we proceed with the instructions, you first need to acquire your dowsing tool, a pendulum. Now, many occult shops sell a pendulum. However, if you are just starting out, you can simply create your own pendulum. All you need is a string or thread, and a needle, the ones used for sewing clothes would be enough. Simply cut the thread to your desired length, about a meter would be enough for a pendulum. Next, tie one end to a needle. You can now use it as a pendulum.

## Chapter 7: Psychic Awareness

Psychic awareness is defined as "the understanding of human consciousness and the full potential of the mind when it is applied to everyday life". Psychic awareness is known to be the understanding of the silent Spirit that lies within us as well as our mind's power. This psychic awareness provides us with access to our subconscious mind, giving us the power to control the various internal energies that influence our health, wellness, and relationships with other people.

There are ways to not only develop but also strengthen your psychic awareness. The power of psychic awareness can then be reapplied to various different areas of our lives. A good way to think of psychic awareness is to think of your brain like a computer. When a computer is unplugged, it can still be used but its uses are greatly limited. When a computer is connected to the internet, however, it has a virtually never-ending list of functions it may perform. When you awaken your Third Eye, it is almost as if you are connecting your brain to the universe's spiritual forces (you then unlock endless possibilities and potential by utilization of your psychic awareness).

We have all heard the science-based rumor that humans only utilize roughly ten percent of our brain's grey matter. Could it be possible that the other untouched 90% deals greatly with psychic awareness? Perhaps through psychic awareness strengthening exercises, and those utilized to achieve Third Eye awakening, we can be able to access and make use of the remaining 90% of our brains.

## Tips to Develop and Strengthen Your Psychic Awareness

1) Pray- Whatever higher power you believe in, whatever religion you practice, ask that higher power to help you have the ability to unlock greater psychic awareness.

2) Meditate- Through meditation, we are able to disconnect from life's general noise and instead form a connection to a deeper awareness of the environment around us as well as our inner selves. When you let go of the preoccupying stressful thoughts you will be able to more easily embrace your mind's natural sense of intuition.

3) Journal- Journaling is a great tool that can help make yourself aware of the external stressors in your life that usually cloud your mind the most. Once you are able to acknowledge these stress factors you can learn when to let go so you may progress moving forward with your Third Eye awakening exercises.

## Chapter 8: Exercises for Awakening Your Inner Spirit

Getting your body moving is one of the best ways to clear your pineal gland and get in touch with your inner spirit. We know that when we exercise, our muscles expand and contract, creating physical movement. What you may not realize is that physical exercise also moves energy around the body. The increase in this energy flow helps you connect your mind and body, as well as your mind and inner spirit.

Any type of physical activity will do. Starting a regular routine consisting of cardiovascular activity like walking or running will get the blood pumping and will keep your heart healthy. Adding weight training will improve strength, preserve bone mass and burn more energy. Any type of activity will raise your body temperature, get your energy flowing and will clear a blocked pineal gland.

There are exercises that focus more on the mind and spirit connection, which may fit better into your overall goals. Practicing yoga is a great place to start. This exercise combines the benefits of strength training and stretching with relaxation and meditation.

If you are not familiar with yoga, it is a guided practice in which specific yoga 'poses' are completed. The movement is generally slow, and the poses are meant to work your muscles and stretch your tendons in a way that would not normally be possible in daily life. You may feel muscles and tendons you didn't know existed after your first class.

Practicing yoga should not be an intimidating task. Although you may be surrounded with other people in a formal class, the idea is to only compete with yourself. Your strength and flexibility will improve with practice, and so you are only trying to improve upon yourself, not compare yourself with others. It is not a game or a competition.

There are many different styles of yoga, ranging from a more regimented class, like Bikram, which uses the same set and combination of poses. Bikram is also often done in a hot room, more than one hundred degrees to add a more cardiovascular component to the practice. This will definitely be too intense for a beginner, but for a seasoned yogi, provides increased flexibility and more spiritual connection. The heat requires the mind to focus exclusively on regulating heart rate and maintaining temperature. With the mind preoccupied on that, it becomes a lot easier to enter a meditative state.

If you are practicing on your own, there are a number of poses to include that will help engage your third eye specifically. Any pose that rests your forehead is benefitting the pineal gland. Mountain pose, in which you bend and rest your forehead on your knees is a great one, although it may take a bit of time to increase your flexibility to this level. Staff pose is similar but a little easier from a seated position. Dolphin pose, a modification of downward dog, is another beginner-level pose. Child's pose is perhaps the easiest of all. The forehead and third eye become grounded to the floor.

More classical meditative yoga is also available, in which the focus is more on the breathing process rather than the physical aspect. Either way, you will be moving your body, increasing energy flow, relaxing and meditating. Yoga is great for helping connect all of your entities, physical, emotional and spiritual. Regular yoga practice will strengthen the body between all three.

Yoga can certainly be a challenge for people who don't move around easily. Although regular practice will improve range of motion, starting with a different type of exercise may be helpful. Practicing Tai Chi is another exercise that has the same meditative properties, but the methods are a bit different.

Tai Chi, although it originated as a form of martial arts, focuses on different poses as well. Instead of being intense and effective for defense, it is a choreographed, graceful movement, constantly flowing from the body. It also focuses on breathing, creating a meditative practice along with the physical exercise. Each pose flows flawlessly into another, with no static pauses, unlike yoga.

Tai Chi is low impact and therefore is open to a greater variety of people. It does not include weight training and does not put a great deal of stress on the cardiovascular system, unlike running or jogging. It is a great practice if you are just beginning an exercise routine. Regular practice has been shown to increase aerobic stamina, increase energy, reduce stress and increased muscle tone.

These benefits are achieved with regular practice, just as with any exercise routine. It is important to maintain a routine to truly feel an improvement in your body and mind. If you are new to Tai Chi, finding a beginners' class is your best bet. Learning the fluidity of the movement takes a bit of practice, but once you get the hang of it, the movement will flow, and you will see more of the meditative benefits.

Regular exercise is mostly about reducing stress when it comes to your third eye. The movement of energy releases tension and increases flow during times of rest. When you are stressed, your body produces stress hormones like cortisol and adrenaline. The goal of these hormones is to raise your heart rate and stimulate muscles to physically flee from danger. This response dates back to the very existence of humans when there was more incidence of physical peril.

These days, our stress comes from late meetings, work schedules and the like. We are not expending the energy given by those hormones, and it builds up, blocking flow within the energy system. Exercise helps relieve some of that tension so that we may be more relaxed overall.

No matter what exercise you decide on, choose something to do regularly that you enjoy. The true benefits of exercise come when you like what you are doing, and you are not just going through the motions. Switch up your exercise routine to keep it interesting, and don't forget to take rest days when your body is feeling fatigued.

## Chapter 9: Pineal Gland Activation and Chakras

### Activation of the Pineal Gland Through Guided Meditation (10-15 Minutes)

The pineal gland is the physical location of the Ajna chakra.

This small pine shaped gland is placed in the middle of the brain.

It controls your sleep cycle, sexual maturation, and many other vital hormones. It produces the DMT, the brain's natural psychedelic drug. It helps us in connecting with our spirituality.

Stimulating this small gland will help you in awakening you spiritually. It will help you in interacting with your divine energies. It will help you in seeing through life.

Start with the breathing exercise.

Inhale slowly, take the fresh air deep into your gut. Gather your worries, tensions, and thoughts.

Now exhale slowly. Release all your worries and tension with the air.

Clear your mind. Racing thoughts are a distraction. You need peace and calm. Soothe your senses. Clear your mind.

Once again, inhale slowly, take the fresh air deep into your gut. Gather your worries, tensions, and thoughts. Now exhale slowly. Release all your worries and tension with the air.

Clear the waste from your mind. Nothing is important at this very moment. You are the prime source of energy. You are embarking on a journey to enlightenment. Start with peace of mind. Tranquility must prevail everywhere.

One more time, inhale slowly, take the fresh air deep into your gut. Gather your worries, tensions, and thoughts. Now exhale slowly. Release all your worries and tension with the air.

Close your eyes and focus.

Focus on the center of your brain. The pineal gland is located here. Establish contact with it. Let it know that you want to connect.

It is very powerful. It is the source of immense power. It is the seat of the soul. The place of the Ajna chakra.

It has spiritual powers. It will help in your unification with the universe. You will become a part of the great network. You do not need an external source. You are the source.

Breathe into the pineal gland. Fill it with divine power. Energize it. You can charge and activate it.

You will feel some throbbing sensation. It is the pineal gland activating.

Focus on it. Let it know that you want to connect with it. You want to become one with your greater self. The eternal light inside you.

Breathe deeply. You want to amalgamate with this divine light. You want to become one with it. Leave all the negative energies behind. Move towards the source of pure and pious energy. The unblemished aura.

It will fill you. It will enlighten you. It will awaken you. Seek and you will find.

Expunge the pollution out of your system. You will not carry anything this point forward. There is no place for worldly feelings. Love, hate, and animosities become meaningless. They create Karma. You are a forgiving soul.

Move ahead. As one with the power. Focus deep. Breathe Deeper.

It is a long journey. Keep moving.

You will feel immense calm. Light all around you. It isn't hot. It is soothing. This is the light of the soul. Your soul is emanating radiance. Absorb it. It is all for you. Relish it.

Enjoy the moment. It is blissful. It is the moment. You have always desired it.

Now, take a deep breath. Inhale slowly, take the fresh air deep into your gut. Wait for a few moments. Now exhale slowly.

Again, take a deep breath. Inhale slowly, take the fresh air deep into your gut. Wait for a few moments. Exhale.

Rub your palms vigorously. Make them warm. Cover your eyes with them. Keep them covered for a moment.

Now open your eyes very slowly. Do not rush. Loosen your body. Do not get up immediately.

Ponder over your achievements in the process.

## Chakras Meaning

Another aspect of spiritual awakening is recognizing and working with the chakra system. Chakras are centers where energy collects throughout the body. They are generally centered around major organ systems, and manipulating the energy and clearing blockages of energy in these areas can help bring more balance to your life and alleviate symptoms associated with a specific chakra.

The chakra system was originally developed in India, centuries ago, and it still plays a major role in Eastern medicine today. Chakras are all about energy balance. Just like your spine, the alignment of your chakras must be just right, or there will be a pain. Learning to pinpoint when a chakra point is out of alignment is the key to fixing it. The body and mind are in a constant state of finding balance. Energy flows and changes, and it is necessary to take stock of your needs, both physical and emotional, as it relates to your chakras, on the regular.

## Types of Chakras

There are seven major chakras in total, all aligned along the centerline of the body. They are as follows:

*Root Chakra:* This energy point is located at the base of the spine, at the tailbone. It is called the root chakra because it is meant to be the energy that grounds you. As you sit on the floor, this chakra is directly in line with the energy of the earth, literally grounding you to it. On a spiritual level, this energy is what keeps you humble and centered in everyday life. It is what gives you purpose, and continually reminds you of your purpose.

A misaligned root chakra can have you feeling as if you are not grounded, unstable. It can manifest itself as having money issues, insecurity finding housing, or a place to call your own. Energy imbalance in this area may lead to trouble securing food or feeling as if you are satisfied. It is associated with the color red.

An imbalance may manifest itself as stiffness in the legs, knee issues, sciatica, a weak immune system, and eating disorders.

*Sacral Chakra:* This chakra gives us the ability to interact and accept others. It is the energy that drives exploration and new experiences. It is located just above the root chakra, about two inches below the navel. Energy from this chakra drives passion and sexual desire, pleasure, and abundance.

A disrupted flow of energy in this chakra can cause a decrease in sex drive, little ability to connect with others on an emotional level and show interest or desire in anything. This chakra is commonly associated with the symptoms of malaise and disinterest during depression. Lack of energy here makes it difficult to show compassion for others and find common ground. It also makes you less able to accept inevitable change in life.

Lack of energy here can manifest itself physically as urinary or sexual issues, kidney problems, and lower back pain.

*Solar Plexus Chakra:* This concentration of energy is centered in the upper abdomen, near the stomach. It is the driving force for our self-confidence and self-esteem. Without this energy, we do not dare to follow through with our goals and aspirations. Without it, we are meek and have no confidence in our capability of success.

Like our pineal gland, the solar plexus helps guide and drive life forward. You may recognize its power as that itch to do something new, to try new things and become more successful. This power waxes and wanes as the chakra moves in and out of alignment. It is associated with the color yellow.

Energy drops may manifest with general fatigue, digestive issues, and gallbladder or pancreas issues, including diabetes.

*Heart Chakra*: It's no surprise that this mass of energy is located on the spine right next to the heart. It is responsible for joy, love and peace. Our heart organ often gets the credit for love, but it is a beaming ray of energy from our heart chakra that fills our chest cavity with feelings of excitement and warmth.

Strengthening this chakra increases our ability and capacity to love, and at what magnitude. It defines the relationships we have and keep. It is associated with the color green, not red, as you might expect!

Issues with respiratory infections, asthma, heart disease and circulatory issues can be a physical manifestation of low energy in the heart chakra.

*Throat Chakra:* This little gem is centered right in the center of our throat. It is responsible for our ability for good communication. When in good alignment, this chakra gives us the energy to articulate our ideas and needs in a way that others can easily understand.

When out of alignment, it may be difficult to work with others and get your point across. We all have moments when it seems like no matter how well you explain something, people don't understand you. Not enough energy is available to formulate your words and emotions in such a way that makes an impact on others.

Issues with the thyroid, laryngitis, ear infections, and shoulder or neck pain are a good indicator that your throat chakra is out of alignment.

*Third Eye Chakra*: Yes, it has its own chakra! It is no wonder that a great mass of energy is centered right where the third eye is located, just above the eyes in the center of your forehead. This chakra is responsible for your intuition and decision-making skills.

You may have felt a decrease in this chakra's energy before, manifested as an inability to make a decision. Generally, wishy-washy people lack energy in this chakra, as their inner self is unable to guide their decisions, leaving them hanging, wondering what to do. Realigning this chakra invites wisdom and confidence that you are making educated decisions.

Chronic headaches, blurry vision, and hormonal imbalance, can all be signs of a third eye energy deficiency. We also cannot forget about depression and anxiety as possible symptoms.

*Crown Chakra:* Last, but not least, the crown chakra represents our ability to be connected spiritually. It is located at the very top of the skull. It represents our ability to see the beauty in the world and have joy within us. As you sit in a seated position, you are rooted in your root chakra, and your spine stands lengthened with your crown chakra pointed straight up to the heavens.

In meditation, this chakra will attract and accept energy in through your head and radiate it throughout your body. Lacking energy in this area means you will find little joy in your surroundings and the rest of your chakras will suffer from lack of energy as well.

Sensitivity to light and sound, as well as depression and the inability to concentrate or learn, are good indications of a problem with your crown chakra.

Knowing the spiritual functions of each chakra makes it easier to pinpoint when anyone is out of alignment. Our bodies and spirits are in a constant state of fluctuation, so at any given time, any chakra may not be functioning properly, even on a day to day basis. It is important to recognize these subtle changes so that adjustments can be made to realign the energy balance.

If one chakra is out of alignment for a long time, it begins to show. For example, if your root chakra is out of whack, you may notice that you lose your ability to control spending, pay bills and keep a secure home. There just isn't enough energy to focus on these things. Over time, the problems mount, creating stress. Aligning this chakra at subtle hints of a problem can help avoid things like financial ruin, loss of relationships or declines in health.

The imbalance of one chakra also causes the overcompensation of others, to try and balance themselves. This can manifest in several ways, depending on which is acting up. You may be doing very well in one aspect of life, but completely failing in another, something many of us recognize. The goal is to balance all energies, so we are strong and successful in all areas of life.

## Sixth Sense – Developing Psychic Awareness

Have you ever had a feeling about something and you just know what others might not feel, or see? Have you ever heard the thoughts of another, but second-guessed that you did? Have you had a dream before that come true days later? Do you ever feel the presence of things that are not of the earthly realm? This is just scratching the surface of some of the things that begin to happen when you awaken your psychic awareness.

As part of Kundalini rising and the process of clearing and releasing blockages and negativity from your subtle body, you shift your perception of reality to the extent that you are able to crack open your latent abilities to receive input from other dimensions. This ability isn't reserved for a select few or passed down genetically through generations, although that has been known to happen. This power to feel beyond the physical realm exists in us all and can be nurtured and grown into everyday use and understanding.

Many people have fear about this level of input because it can feel uncomfortable or vulnerable to tap into the unknown, into things that on the Earth plane we call magic, witchcraft, or superstition. Really, it's truly available to anyone to use this ability. When we are locked in our sleeping state (pre-kundalini rising), we cannot fathom the possibilities of such an existence, but as we allow our awakening to progress fully and reach the state of higher consciousness, we can open the brow and crown chakras to receive and accept our abilities as psychics.

These abilities can manifest in a variety of ways and have been reported as some of the side effects of the awakening process.

# Chapter 10: How to Maintain the Health of Your Third Eye Over Time?

## Steps to Heal Your Third Eye Chakra

Healing your third eye chakra - or any chakra for that matter - is a process. It happens over a gradual succession of healing sessions, and requires your full dedication in order to be considered successful. There are lots of different ways to heal a blocked chakra, but experts often recommend using a combination of methods in order to address an obstruction or poor vibrations.

Before you get started on the actual healing process, it's important that you prepare yourself in order to get the most out of the experience. Being of sound mind, body, and spirit during the healing can help maximize the benefits and remove any barriers that might keep you from experiencing the full power of spiritual healing.

## How to Maximize Your Healing

There are certain factors that act as hindrances towards optimal healing. These are often within our control. Aiming to resolve and eliminate them before we begin any healing methods should improve the outcomes of our practice.

Prepare Your Mind

If this is your first time performing spiritual healing, then you might find yourself questioning the process from start to finish.

"Am I doing this right?"

"Is this the proper execution?"

"I feel silly."

"This probably isn't working."

Stop. These negative thoughts and apprehensions can have an effect on your healing. Your mind is a powerful aspect of your being, and allowing yourself to think these thoughts can create a barrier that prevents positive energy from taking full effect. That's because thinking along these lines is in itself negative energy which works against any positive resonance that might be trying to move into your system.

Before you begin the healing process, try to cleanse your mind. Assure yourself of the benefits of what you're doing and adapt an affirmation to help you absorb the positivity that's coming your way. So instead of telling yourself that it might not be working, focus on the advantages that you've been promised. An example of an affirmation you might want to try can be, "I surrender my negative energy and claim full healing through the powers of the universe."

You can repeat your affirmation to yourself as you go through the healing, especially if you feel that those negative thoughts and apprehensions might be creeping back into your psyche.

Prepare Your Environment

Did you ever notice how you might feel particularly stressed in a space that's cluttered or dirty? Regardless of our unique standards when it comes to cleanliness and orderliness, certain environmental conditions can cause significant distress, making us feel out of sorts, anxious, and unhappy.

In the same way, you shouldn't attempt any sort of healing in a space that doesn't resonate with your soul. Dirty, cluttered rooms can vibrate negative energy, causing any positive resonance from being fully absorbed. That's why it's important to make sure you've fully prepared a space to help maximize your healing.

What are the factors that make up a prepared environment?

A comfortable place to sit or to lie down, depending on the healing method you've chosen. Always seek a set-up that lets you assume straight posture as this can help improve the flow of energy.

If you're sitting, it's always best to ditch the chair and sit on the floor instead. Lay down a clean yoga mat or a pillow and make sure you can sit up straight. For methods that require you to lie down, always opt for a slight recline at around 30-45 degrees.

Dim lights help draw attention away from what's seen and improve your ability to zone in on your mentality. Darkness also helps soothe the body, allowing a calmer disposition that's ideal for healing. Dim down the lights just enough for you to make out the items inside a space, but not enough to be engulfed in complete darkness.

Music can be a great way to maintain focus because complete silence - contrary to popular belief - can actually turn into a distraction and may keep your mind from fully entering the meditative state. That's because your mind needs constant external stimulation, which is why silence might make you feel uneasy or restless.

Instead of playing traditional music though, you may want to experiment with other sounds. Calm chiming sounds are often a great choice for beginners. There are also audio files of natural sounds that you can use, such as the sounds of flowing water and wind rustling through trees.

Involving your sense of smell can also help improve the healing process. Certain fragrances - especially those from essential oils - can positively impact the brain and trigger the release of chemicals in the brain to achieve a happier, more proactive mentality.

Some of the best essential oils for meditation and chakra healing include frankincense, lavender, peppermint, sandalwood, and ylang-ylang. Diffuse a small amount using an essential oil diffuser and allow the scent to completely engulf your space before you begin the process.

Essentially, a prepared environment for healing is a space that engages all of your senses. Because we're all different, our preferences may have an effect on what we feel to be the best environment for chakra healing. However, by utilizing these tips, you should be able to come up with the optimal set-up so you can achieve the most with each session.

Prepare Your Body

Stimulation coming from your body can impact your healing session negatively. For instance, the urge to relieve yourself can interfere with your thoughts, distracting you from your goal. Hunger, sleepiness, and discomfort are all potential interferences that can cut your healing short.

Make sure your body is prepared for the process before you begin. Relieve yourself, take a shower, and make sure you've eaten enough food to satiate your hunger. Stay hydrated and keep a cup of water close to you to quench your thirst should it become an issue during the healing.

In terms of comfort, the way you prepare your environment will play a major role. Always make sure to try out your set-up before you engage in the process to identify any possible noxious stimuli that could distract you. It also helps to schedule your session for after you wake up in the morning or from a nap so you don't end up feeling too sleep to successfully heal your chakra.

Tools and Resources for Healing the Third Eye

Did you know that each chakra corresponds to unique objects and substances in our environment? This happens because each unique item and material resonates with a specific energy signature that may vibrate more closely to certain energy centers. Focusing on using the items, tools, and resources that resonate with your third eye can help make healing much more beneficial.

Food for the Third Eye

Achieving a balance of the third eye may require that you indulge in foods that exhibit a purple hue. Always focus on naturally colored foods, and not choices that might be purple by use of food coloring or artificial ingredients.

Here are some foods that might be able to resonate best with your third eye:

Eggplants

Grapes

Blackberries or mulberries

Purple kale

Purple cabbage

Onions

Purple yams

Similarly, there are other non-purple food choices that might be beneficial for third eye healing as well. These include natural cacao and foods rich in omega-3. These foods are said to boost brain power, allowing them to tap into the third eye to achieve balance and reveal this chakra's unique powers.

Aside from incorporating these ingredients into your daily diet, you may want to indulge in a pre-healing snack that uses one or more of these ingredients. This can help fuel the third eye to make it more responsive to your healing techniques.

Crystals for the Third Eye

There are over a thousand different kinds of crystals, and each one offers unique benefits for the mystic healer. But if you were hoping to specifically address your third eye, then you may want to consider investing in stones that are known to help address the Ajna chakra.

These include:

Amethyst

Angelite

Azurite

Fluorite

Iolite

Labradorite

Moonstone

Crystals can be used for a variety of healing techniques, including wearing, placing, swinging, and grids. Using these crystals for any one of these techniques and endowing them with the right intention to address the third eye can be especially beneficial.

Other Tools to Heal the Third Eye

The third eye chakra uses the element of light. This energy center casts light on dark areas of the mind to help you see ideas, thoughts, emotions, and circumstances through new 'eyes'. By illuminating these concepts with its spiritual rays of light, your third eye gives you perspectives anew, allowing you greater intuition, empathy, and intellect.

That said, you should know that the third eye responds strongly to natural sources of light. Sunlight and moonlight are both powerful tools that you can leverage to help your third eye resonate with the right vibrations. It also helps to stargaze, allowing you to absorb the subtle energy of distant sources of powerful light around us.

Remember that the chakras are not isolated energy centers, but interconnected ganglion of vibrations. Energy passes from chakra to chakra, so a disturbance in the resonance of one chakra can have an impact on others. In the case of the third eye, any issues you may experience relative to this 6th chakra might actually be the result of an obstruction in another chakra - especially the root chakra.

Establishing a groundedness and security through your root chakra can help resolve a variety of problems that you might be experiencing elsewhere. If you find that you have an obstruction in your root chakra, address that before anything else. It might be causing the rest of the spiritual, physical, emotional, and mental disturbances you're feeling.

Finally, the third eye chakra is one of the most creative energy centers in your system. The more you stimulate creativity, the more your third eye becomes enriched with positive vibrations. Find a creative activity that resonates with your mind and soul - like painting, sculpting, or sketching. Some people enjoy writing, singing, and playing an instrument, which are all suitable channels for creative expression.

Establishing a Healing Regimen

Our chakras can become routinely blocked because we're never completely free from the effects of negative vibrations. An unhappy coworker, stressful conditions at home, school, or work, problems in our relationships, poor food choices, environmental noise, and everything in between - all of these stressors can impose negative resonance on our chakras.

So, it's important to make sure you heal your third eye regularly, even if you don't sense too significant of a blockage. Here's a sample routine you can implement in your lifestyle to address any issues with the spinning movement of your third eye:

Incorporate third eye enriching foods into at least one meal every day.

Create an energy grid an bestow an intention for third eye health. Keep it active for at least 1 week every month.

Wear a third eye crystal like amethyst as an amulet daily. You can also keep a small tumbled stone in your pocket to grasp and hold if you feel the need to fight off negative energies.

Once a month, meditate on your spiritual energy. If you sense any factors that might be hindering your third eye from being fully active, sever that energy cord.

Try to work in at least 1 hour of creative work 2 days a week. You can mix up your technique by interchanging activities to keep your interest and creative energy up.

Increasing the Efficiency of Your 3rd Eye through Clairvoyance

What would you say clairvoyance is? Well, according to the plain English meaning it is that ability to perceive things in an extraordinary way; having a peep into the future which is not equivalent to wishing – rather, some sensory feel of the reality to come.

With reference to the power of the third eye, you are a clairvoyant when you can see something beforehand – meaning a real view of some future happening; see something happening in real time even when you are not close enough to apply your five common senses; and even visualizing something that happened sometime in the past even when you were not privy to it.

Now, have we just said that a clairvoyant can tell the reality pertaining to the past; now; and the future without hearing, seeing, touching, smelling or even feeling? Right! And you may be thinking – those must be the queer looking ladies whose appointments are shrouded in mystery and secrecy; whose fees you pay through the nose. But no – not always... Whereas clairvoyance is a unique practice, it is not because it is a preserve of a few. And clairvoyants need not look weird, scary or funny. Of course, I'll spice it a little bit with some aura of mystery if I'm charging you the services; just to play on your psychology, but really, clairvoyance is something you can also learn, practice and master.

Let us try and understand how the powers of a clairvoyant manifest:

Having a dream that is vivid and then whatever was in the dream comes to pass.

Misplacing something you had and then while you are just mum a mental picture of the place you put the thing flashes through your mind – and the thing happened to be right where your mental image took you.

You could be driving and then you mentally see the actual car you are following turning, say, to the right; and in a minute or so, it literally does so.

You see someone's image mentally – what sometimes we mistake for 'thinking' about someone; and sometime later in the day that same person gets in touch with you, either in person or via phone or even mail.

Supposing you could do that on all important matters! Yet it is possible for you to enhance the natural power of clairvoyance that you may currently have in your own small way, and be able to visualize things in a more mentally intense manner.

Here are some steps you can take in enhancing your power of clairvoyance:

Abandon your fears

Have you been in a situation where you were so scared of something or someone and had to laugh about it later when you got accustomed to them? I'm imagining being born and brought up on an island where tortoises and turtles were about the only animals you saw. Then one day someone flew you out to the tropics where you saw herds of 4 – 5 meter tall giraffes. You would think it was not real but a figment of your imagination!

That is the same thing that happens particularly when you are young and you get clairvoyant experiences. If they are scary compared to your situation in real life, you chuck it aside so you will not have to deal with the truth.

Such is the scenario when a kid has a clairvoyant experience of her or his parents parting ways in a divorce

A child also shuts out clairvoyant experiences if parents or other adults attribute narrations of such experiences as evil

A child can also shut out such clairvoyant experiences when mature people fail to believe them and accuse them of lying or having an exaggerated imagination

So what is the reality for the child? The truth is that a child may be born with the third eye clearly open and with clairvoyant abilities very strong, and may, therefore, be seeing his or her spiritual guides very vividly and having clairvoyant experiences with clarity.

How, then, do you rid yourself of this limiting fear?

You can release the fear that inhibits your ability to perceive things as per your natural abilities by affirming your belief in yourself.

Get a place to sit and make yourself comfortable

While relaxed, take two or even three long, deep breaths

As you do the inhaling and exhaling, say something like this: I'm prepared to let go of all the fear that I have of seeing into the future.

Be sincere in your questioning

Sometimes you want to use your clairvoyant abilities in a conscious way and so you pose a question to your inner self – be genuine and to the point. It is the only way you are going to receive an answer that is accurate and helpful to you. In short, the reason you are applying your clairvoyance is that you have genuine curiosity and desires. Express them as you feel them.

If, for instance, you are longing to find a romantic partner at a particular party, design your question as precisely as you can, like:

Shall I meet a romantic partner at the party tonight? Or:

Shall I get involved with someone romantically tonight?

The point is to avoid being vague like:

I'm I likely to meet someone?

Think about it this way. If you ask vaguely and get the answer in the affirmative, you could end up meeting a long lost relative or a very interesting comic. Yes! In both cases you will have met someone. But is it the kind of person you are longing for? No. So be to the point and give details as close as you can; otherwise you may end up doubting your clairvoyance while it is your questioning technique that is wanting.

Further Enhancement of Your 3rd Eye through Clairvoyance

Do you recall why you are so interested in applying your clairvoyance? It is because you are curious about something you deem important, like the possibility of you linking up with a romantic partner. So, this is what you do to help get clear answers:

Direct your total focus on your third eye

Sit down and relax

Direct your focus on your 6th chakra

Sixth. Yes – that chakra that resides just between your eyes and slightly above; between your eyebrows, to be precise. That one is in charge of your high level intuition. That is the position of your third eye, which experts call Ajna, and which is known to discharge sharp sensory messages that are clear and telling. As usual, you are taking deep breaths as you concentrate on your third eye – three ins and outs will suffice.

What you are essentially working on is getting this intense energy center that is your 6th chakra to activate your clairvoyance, and hence begin sending psychic images in response to your questions.

And will you get them?

Well, first ascertain that you can see some oval shape (eyelike) at the place where the chakra is supposed to be.

Now, is that eyelike shape closed?

Or is it partially open?

Is it clearly open?

The point is you want that eyelike shape clearly open because that is your third eye, the facilitator of clairvoyance. In case it is not yet open, you need to repeat your affirmation that you are actually prepared to discard all your fears associated with psychic sight; that you are eager to see psychically.

Do you know how you will tell that your third eye has finally opened up besides visualizing it on the oval shape?

You will suddenly enjoy a calming feeling of warm engulfing love.

Take note of the pictures entering your mind

And how do I monitor those pictures, you may be wondering? This is what you need to look out for:

A picture lingering in your mind in singular – one vivid image

A picture lingering before your eyes in singular – again one unmistakable picture

A movie-like image shows within your mind; within your mental arena

A movie-like image shows before your eyes; beyond your mental arena

And what colors do these pictures come in?

These images do not come in pre-defined colors despite the fact that the third eye is linked to Color Purple or Indigo.

They sometimes come in plain black and white

Other times the images come in a full range of colors

There are times that you see the images in form of cartoons

Other times you may even see an image in form of a distinct painting

Seek to enhance the brightness as well as the size of your psychic images

How do you do that? Simple: commanding affirmation! With conviction and belief you address your mental pictures in this manner:

My pictures, I direct you to grow in size as well as strength right away!

The idea is to communicate clearly:

Your unequivocal decision to venture into the realm of the psychic

Your undivided attention to the emerging images

Your strong intention to embrace those psychic images

And with that declaration, your pictures become more pronounced – larger; bolder; and even brighter – in a way that is relatively easy to decipher. We have said that this is going to work and it surely should, and you need to believe too that it will.

But supposing there seems to be a hitch with the clarity of the images still not very helpful?

Please note that you will not be the first person to whose first attempt was not exactly yielding.

Seek interpretation as well as clarification

What is the use of seeing an image if you cannot tell what it represents? Unless you can derive meaning from the pictures that you see in your mind, you will still remain as uninformed as that person with no interest in psychic powers – or even more confused.

Therefore, address the powers in your spiritual world thus:

What is the meaning of these images?

And you can ask that mentally or even verbally, it does not matter. Have faith in your spiritual powers because your guides in the spiritual world are actually intent on helping you; they are normally very co-operative.

Maintain your quiet concentration and you will be rewarded with clear answers in form of:

Feeling

Sound

Thought

Any of those three could be the form in which you get your response.

If you really do not comprehend your answer as communicated, address your spiritual powers and request that you be sent the answers again in a form that you can easily understand.

Maintain your trust

It is just like in your normal day-to-day activities. How can you succeed if you are working with a system that you do not believe in; a system you hardly trust? Impossible! So, in these matters of clairvoyance, doubting the strength or credibility of the psychic system is sure self-sabotage. You must trust what you are working with – your psychic ability; your clairvoyance; your ability to get answers pertaining to your future. It is absolutely crucial that you believe and trust in the clairvoyant images that you receive too. That way, they are going to work as expected as there are no conflicting energies.

# Chapter 11: Common Mistakes People Make Trying to Activate the Third Eye

If there is something worse than not doing something, then it is doing it in the wrong way. The same is true for third eye activation. If you are trying to awaken your third eye and doing it incorrectly, then you are up for some pretty bad experiences. Third eye awakening is a powerful practice that must be done carefully and with great dedication.

If you are looking for quick results or instant gratification, then you will be stepping in the wrong realm. Some people keep trying but never have any luck with their third eye activation. It isn't that the third eye is not present in them, it seems that they are improperly looking for something. Not understanding the signs or misinterpreting them can also lead to failure or desperation.

The following are some of the mistakes people make while trying to activate their third eye. You must avoid them.

Indulging in Misinformation

TV, media, and internet are great tools for spreading misinformation. They have a knack for making a mountain of a molehill. They can make you believe absurd things that may lead to desperation in the end. Before you begin your third eye activation, you must make yourself aware of the things you are going to encounter on your way. Do not expect too much or too little. Judging the gap always prevents falling in it. Do your homework properly before you embark on the journey of activating your third eye.

Lack of Trust

Trust is a very important factor when you go on any journey, especially the ones involving adventure. Third eye activation is an adventure trip like you have never taken. To experience it, you must have trust in yourself and your instincts. You must not distrust anything that you see or feel while you are trying to activate your third eye. You must also give proper importance to the changes you experience on the way. Remaining conscious of even the smallest of events is very important.

Lack of Purpose

People who lack a clear purpose for activating their third eye will face failures. Activating the third eye is not a walk in the park. You can't shake it off as you do with other things. It starts some irreversible processes. You must have a definite purpose for activating the third eye. Only then will you be able to judge the amount of success you have achieved in your pursuits. If you are not looking for something specific, you may not find anything at all.

Lack of Technique

Following a proper technique is very important for activating the third eye. Third eye activation may look like an undefined path. The journey inside doesn't have a definite route, but using the right technique is very important or you can start feeling lost. Pick a technique that suits you the best, and please follow it carefully. Do not keep changing your methods or you may not achieve anything at all. Remain regular in your practice and do it with great devotion. People who take this lightly end up wasting their time.

Trying too hard

Do not try too hard. Those who want quick success often start trying too hard in the beginning. It may lead to desperation or your mind will start cooking up false stories, and both will lead to failure. When trying to activate your third eye, focus on the technique and let things happen on their own. Do not try to force your mind to think in a particular way or imagine things. Overdependence on visualization will lead to the framing of false notions in your mind. You may start viewing things that you want to see without having achieved anything at all.

Stop Looking for the Wrong Signs

You must look for the right signs. Some so-called experts have attached some wrong notions with the third eye activation method. They have made people believe that third eye activation will only happen if they get specific signs. This is inaccurate. Look for the subtle changes taking place inside you. Trust your instincts and take a lead. Do not go by the wrong notions. Your experience with third eye awakening may be totally different than others. If you keep looking for the experiences of others you may never feel satisfied.

No Instant Results

Third eye activation is not similar to ordering anything on the internet. It doesn't happen instantaneously. Even after your third eye has awakened, you may not be able to see a significant change for a very long time. Honing your abilities takes much longer than that and requires a lot of practice. You must pay great attention to this aspect.

Not Enough Practice

You will need to practice your skills for quite some time to have measurable results. Even if your third eye is active, it will not give you significant results if you fail to practice it regularly. You have to train your mind to look in the right direction. Your mind must learn to recognize the signs. It must learn to look at things with better insight. All this will only happen when you practice regularly. Make meditation a part of your schedule. Do not miss it or give excuses to yourself. By doing so, you'll only be bringing failure to your pursuit.

Avoid Overpublicizing Your Efforts

The journey to awaken your third eye is a personal quest. It is a long journey, and the ride is never smooth. You must avoid talking about it to your friends. Such discussions spark negative criticism and envy. You may start getting labeled or ridiculed, and it may lead to doubts. Keep it to yourself, and keep practicing. It is one of the best ways to preserve your positive energies and get better results.

## Conclusion

In the beginning, many people want simple meditation techniques. Some types of meditation that are good for beginners are brain wave meditation, breathing meditation, or hypnotic meditation. The third eye (related to the sixth chakra) is a known property of the etheric body. It contains numerous psychic powers of higher consciousness, including clairvoyance and ESP. Recent research is increasingly converging on the possible connection between the third eye and the pineal gland, which is a unique part of the brain because it is not directly connected to either hemisphere. Subsequent studies have now provided conclusive evidence of the adverse effects of fluoride on the pineal gland. In the interest of developing human awareness, it is essential to nourish the pineal gland and prevent inorganic contaminants from irreversibly damaging this critical part of the brain.

Opening your heart is an indication of literally opening your physical heart to the frequency of real love, which is unconditional love. It is a self-love that is not based on ego needs, recognition, or worldly achievements. When you open your physical heart, you open your chakra heart, and that makes love flow through your brain, your body, and the whole world. It is an authentic life. Most people think they feel real love when they are in love or in a relationship. This may be the case for a few, but the majority of people assume anxiety, depression, cynicism, internal violence, and lack of self-compassion, so they really start from conditional love. When you give love to receive love, you are in a conditioned relationship.

The laws of attraction always direct your mind and your life towards wellbeing. This flow is blocked when you stop accepting things as they come. If you learn to accept good or bad things, you will find that all things lead to a better part of yourself. To expand your mind, you need to be more open to things. Being open to things can be different than you previously imagined. When you expand your mind, things that you would like to bring to yourself become sooner than that you pursue them. The majority of people have no clue how it works.

Meditation techniques could help you deal with today's life, which is full of struggles and stress. If you choose to slow down, there is a good chance that it will be left behind. Most of us live a stressful life and are overloaded with work to keep up with others. Stress is the gateway to all mental and emotional complaints. Meditation is the best way to relieve stress and live a healthy and happy life. Meditation is traditionally done with the focus on objects like a candle or your breath. Through meditation, mind, and body relax, and you experience inner peace. The more concentrated you are, the better results you will get. Meditation helps develop your level of concentration. Many people among us believe that meditation is not for us and cannot work in our situation. Well, this is completely wrong, and the fact is that anyone can learn meditation easily, and if you practice it regularly, it will help you to know yourself better.

By **Spiritual Awakening Academy**

www.ingramcontent.com/pod-product-compliance
Lightning Source LLC
Chambersburg PA
CBHW050248120526
44590CB00016B/2259